Multiple Myeloma

Remedica State of the Art series
ISSN 1472-4626

Also available
Handbook of Diabetes Mellitus and Cardiovascular Disease
The Inflammatory Bowel Disease Yearbook 2003
Kidney Transplantation
Management of Atherosclerotic Carotid Disease
Management of Peripheral Arterial Disease
Rheumatoid Arthritis
Viral Co-infections in HIV: Impact and Management

Published by Remedica Publishing
32–38 Osnaburgh Street, London, NW1 3ND, UK
20 N Wacker Drive, Suite 1642, Chicago, IL, USA

E-mail: books@remedica.com
www.remedica.com

Publisher: Andrew Ward
In-house editors: Emma Hawkridge, James Griffin

ISBN 1 901346 48 X
British Library Cataloguing-in Publication Data
A catalogue record for this book is available from the British Library

Multiple Myeloma

Editors

Paul G Richardson

Assistant Professor of Medicine, Harvard Medical School
Clinical Director, Jerome Lipper Multiple Myeloma Center
Division of Hematologic Oncology
Dana-Farber Cancer Institute
44 Binney Street
Boston, MA 02115
USA

Kenneth C Anderson

Kraft Family Professor of Medicine, Harvard Medical School
Director, Jerome Lipper Multiple Myeloma Center
Division of Hematologic Oncology
Dana-Farber Cancer Institute
44 Binney Street
Boston, MA 02115
USA

REMEDICA
publishing

LONDON • CHICAGO

Contributors

Melissa Alsina, MD
Assistant Professor, Department of Interdisciplinary Oncology,
H Lee Moffitt Cancer Center & Research Institute,
12902 Magnolia Drive, Tampa, FL 33612, USA

P Leif Bergsagel, MD
Associate Professor of Medicine, Weill Medical College of
Cornell University, Department of Medicine, New York
Presbyterian Hospital, 1300 York Avenue, Room C609,
New York, NY 10021, USA

Jamie D Cavenagh, MD, FRCP, MRCPath
Senior Lecturer (Honorary Consultant) in Haematology,
St Bartholomew's Hospital, West Smithfield,
London EC1A 7BE, UK

Peter I Croucher, MD
Senior Research Fellow, Nuffield Department of Orthopaedic
Surgery, Nuffield Orthopaedic Centre, Windmill Road,
Oxford OX3 7LD, UK

Teru Hideshima, MD, PhD
Principal Associate, Harvard Medical School, Jerome Lipper
Multiple Myeloma Center, Division of Hematologic Oncology,
Dana-Farber Cancer Institute, 44 Binney Street, Boston,
MA 02115, USA

Sundar Jagannath, MD
Chief, Multiple Myeloma Service, Bone Marrow and Blood Stem
Cell Transplantation, St. Vincent's Comprehensive Cancer
Center, 325 West 15th Street, New York, NY 10011, USA

Robert A Kyle, MD
Professor of Medicine and Laboratory Medicine, Mayo Medical School, Consultant, Division of Hematology, Mayo Clinic, 200 First Street SW, Rochester, MN 55905, USA

Nikhil C Munshi, MD
Associate Director, Jerome Lipper Multiple Myeloma Center, Division of Hematologic Oncology, Dana-Farber Cancer Institute, 44 Binney Street, Boston, MA 02115, USA

S Vincent Rajkumar, MD
Associate Professor of Medicine, Mayo Medical School, Consultant, Division of Hematology, Mayo Clinic, 200 First Street SW, Rochester, MN 55905, USA

Robert L Schlossman, MD
Instructor in Medicine, Harvard Medical School, Jerome Lipper Multiple Myeloma Center, Division of Hematologic Oncology, Dana-Farber Cancer Institute, 44 Binney Street, Boston, MA 02115, USA

Kenneth H Shain, PhD
Researcher, Department of Interdisciplinary Oncology, H Lee Moffitt Cancer Center & Research Institute, 12902 Magnolia Drive, Tampa, FL 33612, USA

Donna M Weber, MD
Assistant Professor, The University of Texas MD Anderson Cancer Center, 1515 Holcombe Blvd, Box 429, Houston, TX 77030, USA

To our wonderful wives, Annie and Cynthia, and our children, Faith, Edward, William, Emily, David, and Peter, whose support has been invaluable both in our work and during preparation of this book.

PGR, KCA

Foreword

While multiple myeloma comes under the definition of an "orphan disease", more than 45,000 individuals live with this illness in the USA alone, and approximately 14,000 Americans are diagnosed each year. The first descriptions of myeloma were documented in the mid-1840s, and not until the discovery of sarcolysin in Russia in 1958 was a promising therapy developed. From sarcolysin, melphalan was derived, and in 1962 Daniel Bergsagel described the first successful use of this drug for the treatment of myeloma. Pioneer investigators of the disease, including Sydney Salmon and Raymond Alexanian, introduced the use of prednisone, and in 1969 Alexanian demonstrated that the combination of melphalan plus prednisone was superior to melphalan alone. These discoveries definitely improved the survival time and wellbeing of many patients with multiple myeloma, but, unfortunately, these drugs cured few, if any, patients.

Almost four decades later, the use of melphalan and prednisone remains the mainstay for treatment of many patients with multiple myeloma, and the median survival time has not dramatically improved from the 3–4 years described in the 1970s. And yet there is hope and even optimism that this will soon change, and that newly discovered treatments will result in improved overall survival time and quality of life.

In this well-written book edited and compiled by Paul Richardson and Kenneth Anderson, a concise description by Bergsagel of the epidemiology and molecular pathogenesis of multiple myeloma lays the groundwork for the authors of subsequent chapters, who describe the novel therapies that are being developed to target specific and unique molecular pathways involved in the oncogenesis of myeloma. The assumption is that targeting these unique molecular pathways will result in more effective and less toxic therapies and, perhaps eventually, a curative approach. The first chapter describes genetic abnormalities that may be involved in the etiology of myeloma. Furthermore, the discovery of the genetic origins of the disease may explain racial differences in the incidence of myeloma, and these discoveries may ultimately lead to actual prevention or at least a halting of progression of the plasma cell neoplasms at an early stage of the disease. Hopefully the newly discovered molecular oncogenic mechanisms associated with multiple myeloma will provide novel approaches to preventing disease progression and dealing with morbid problems such as osteolysis and bone damage.

Since the discovery of melphalan, numerous other cytotoxic agents have been used in the treatment of myeloma; however, various combinations of these agents have done little to improve overall survival time compared with melphalan and prednisone. The use of high-dose cytotoxics, especially melphalan, has improved survival time compared with standard doses of cytotoxics, but even this approach ultimately leads to drug resistance and death due to progressive disease. Therefore, the development of drug resistance in multiple myeloma is considered a major obstacle to curing this disease. In Chapter 2, Shain and Alsina describe two different types of drug-resistant phenotypes that result in disease progression. The best-described form of resistance is an acquired resistance that is intrinsically related to genetic adaptation of the myeloma cell, and has been given the term multidrug resistance, or MDR. Several different molecular mechanisms have been associated with this form of resistance, and attempts to circumvent MDR have not, so far, been successful. A newer and more transient form of drug resistance is associated with the tumor microenvironment and may be considered a form of *de novo* drug resistance. Interactions between myeloma cells and bone marrow stromal cells appear to create a survival advantage for the myeloma cells and reduce drug treatment activity. Perhaps addressing this *de novo* form of drug resistance by targeting the microenvironment may enhance the effects of drugs and improve patient outcome.

In fact, Chapter 3, by Richardson, Hideshima, and Anderson, looks at novel therapies that attack not only the myeloma cell but also target the tumor microenvironment, ultimately resulting in the death of the myeloma cell. Potential targets include certain soluble cytokines, including interleukin-6 and vascular endothelial growth factor (VEGF). These new agents include thalidomide and immunomodulatory drugs, the proteasome inhibitor bortezomib, VEGF inhibitors, and an array of other drugs that target unique signaling pathways associated with tumor–host cell interactions. In the past decade, a virtual information explosion has occurred regarding our understanding of the molecular pathogenesis of multiple myeloma, and fortunately a vast array of new drugs is being developed that target these novel pathways. Never before have so many new drug choices been available for study in multiple myeloma patients. This excitement is further enhanced by the new approach to drug development, which now involves a target-based rationale, replacing the previous blind empiricism of combining various cytotoxics.

In Chapter 4, Weber focuses on the use of thalidomide as a novel treatment for multiple myeloma and, in her excellent review, provides evidence that thalidomide (probably in combination with dexamethasone) may actually replace the mainstay of melphalan plus prednisone in newly diagnosed patients. No treatment is without side effects, however, and since the initial description of thalidomide in 1999, a number of side effects have been described. Other issues include establishing the most effective and least toxic dose of thalidomide, combining thalidomide with other agents, and the best point during the course of the disease to use the drug.

Perhaps the most profound new approach to treating myeloma that has resulted in improved overall survival time is the use of high-dose chemotherapy (HDT) combined with stem cell rescue.

Melphalan at high doses appears to be the most effective cytotoxic agent, and was first described by McElwain and Powles in the early 1980s. Munshi, Schlossman, and Jagannath provide an excellent description of the evidence supporting the use of HDT; however, many questions still remain, including the timing of therapy during the course of disease, tandem versus single high-dose treatments, use of maintenance therapy following HDT, and the role of allogeneic transplantation. The evidence to date, however, is compelling enough in support of HDT that transplant-appropriate patients with multiple myeloma should at least consider it as a treatment option.

Another advance that has definitely improved the quality of life of multiple myeloma patients is the treatment of myeloma-associated bone disease. Cavenagh and Croucher provide an outstanding description of the normal process of bone marrow remodeling and the dysfunction that occurs in this process due to multiple myeloma, resulting in bone destruction. The discussion of the use of bisphosphonate therapy is particularly informative and addresses some of the transatlantic biases in the use of oral versus intravenous bisphosphonates. A very clear comparison is made between the guidelines established in the UK and those recommended by the American Society of Clinical Oncology. Perhaps as we gain a greater understanding of the complex mechanisms associated with myeloma-related bone destruction, new targets for therapeutic intervention will be identified and the transatlantic debate over which bisphosphonate is more effective will become mute.

Finally, Chapter 7, by Rajkumar and Kyle, is particularly useful in addressing the individual patient with multiple myeloma. Beginning by describing the appropriate criteria for diagnosing multiple myeloma, the authors provide very useful and practical approaches to the treatment and follow-up of newly diagnosed patients. The vast experience of Dr Kyle allows him to almost anticipate the questions of practitioners who encounter various problems experienced by patients at various stages of their disease.

This chapter does more than just discuss treatment options; it appears to synthesize an approach that considers most of the challenges and dilemmas that face both the patient and physician caring for the patient. Importantly, this chapter also deals with common but troublesome problems such as supportive care measures and pain management.

Although multiple myeloma remains an incurable disease to date, never before has there been such justified enthusiasm and optimism about the research and treatment of this disease. Translational research is alive and well in capitalizing on the discoveries of the pathogenesis of myeloma for developing target-based therapies that are truly novel and, hopefully, have improved effectiveness and reduced toxicity. *Carpe diem*!

William Dalton, MD
Professor, Associate Center Director for Clinical Investigations/
Chairman, Interdisciplinary Oncology Program/Deputy Director/
Professor of Oncology, Medicine and Biochemistry,
H Lee Moffitt Cancer Center & Research Institute, FL, USA

About the Editors

Paul G Richardson, MD

Dr Richardson received his MD from the Medical College of St Bartholomew's Hospital, University of London, and part of his residency training at the Royal Marsden Hospital, London and Sutton. After a clinical fellowship at Baystate Medical Center of Tufts University School of Medicine, he joined the Dana-Farber Cancer Institute, MA, USA, and spent 5 years with the Solid Tumor Autologous Marrow Program, also completing a medical residency at Beth Israel Hospital during that time. He joined Dr Kenneth Anderson at the Jerome Lipper Multiple Myeloma Center in 1999, becoming its Clinical Director in 2001. He is board certified in internal medicine, hematology, and medical oncology, and is an Assistant Professor of Medicine at Harvard Medical School. His primary research interests are novel, biologically derived therapies for multiple myeloma, and new treatments for regimen-related toxicities occurring during bone marrow and stem cell transplantation.

Kenneth C Anderson, MD

Dr Anderson graduated from Johns Hopkins Medical School, MD, USA, trained in internal medicine at Johns Hopkins Hospital, and completed hematology, medical oncology, and tumor immunology training at the Dana-Farber Cancer Institute, MA, USA. He is the Kraft Family Professor of Medicine at Harvard Medical School, and serves as Chief of the Division of Hematologic Neoplasia, Director of the Jerome Lipper Multiple Myeloma Center, and Vice Chair of the Joint Program in Transfusion Medicine at Dana-Farber Cancer Institute. His translational research focuses on the development of novel therapeutics targeting the myeloma cell in its microenvironment. He hosted the VI International Myeloma Workshop on Multiple Myeloma, serves on the Board of Directors and as Chairman of the Scientific Advisors of the Multiple Myeloma Research Foundation, and is a Doris Duke Distinguished Clinical Research Scientist. In 2003, he received the Waldenstrom's Award for his research into plasma cell dyscrasias.

Preface

Significant advances in our understanding of the biology of multiple myeloma (MM) have led to exciting new opportunities for treatment. The successful translation of these derived novel therapies from laboratory bench to bedside, with less toxicity and more specific anti-MM activity, has engendered new hope for improved patient outcome.

This book provides a concise overview of the present state of the art relating to MM biology and therapy. We hope that it will thus give readers, be they specialist hematologist/oncologists, generalists, or other interested healthcare providers – including those in training – a comprehensive but concise overview of MM biology and treatment, and provide insight into the exciting future of therapeutic opportunities for this hitherto deadly illness.

We are grateful to all of the contributors for their expert work in condensing the current knowledge regarding the background, treatment, and management of multiple myeloma, and turning it into a clearly-written review of the state of the art in this therapeutic area. We would also like to thank Remedica, the publisher, for editorial and design support, and for making this book possible.

Paul G Richardson
Kenneth C Anderson

Contents

1

Epidemiology, etiology, and molecular pathogenesis

P Leif Bergsagel

Introduction

Multiple myeloma (MM) is a malignant plasma cell tumor that is distributed at multiple sites within the bone marrow (BM) compartment. It accounts for approximately 12,000 deaths per year in the US alone [1]. The incidence is twofold higher in American blacks than whites, with a significantly higher incidence in males for each population. The roles of genetic background and environment are poorly defined, though there is suggestive evidence of some clustering within families [2].

Stages of multiple myeloma

Plasma cell neoplasms are distinguished by an idiotypic rearrangement of the immunoglobulin (Ig) gene, which occurs prior to the malignant transformation of a plasma cell precursor. The clone that develops must increase to about 5×10^9 cells before it produces enough of the idiotypic Ig for a monoclonal (M) "spike" to be recognized in a serum electrophoresis pattern.

Most subjects with a serum M protein are asymptomatic. If other causes of an M protein can be ruled out, the condition is labeled as monoclonal gammopathy of undetermined significance (MGUS). By definition, the clone in MGUS is stable, and the serum M protein concentration remains level for many years. However, prolonged follow-up of a large group of MGUS subjects has shown that, every year, about 2% of these patients develop symptomatic MM, macroglobulinemia, malignant lymphoma, chronic lymphocytic leukemia, or amyloidosis [3]. MGUS is considered to be a premalignant lesion because the clone does not grow progressively; it is stable and asymptomatic.

Almost all of the genetic aberrations identified in MM (aneuploidy, monosomy 13, and 14q32 chromosome translocations) are also present in MGUS [4]. Additional neoplastic changes are required to convert this large, stable clone into a progressively expanding tumor with malignant characteristics – ie, MM. MM is distinguished from MGUS by having a greater intramedullary tumor cell content (>10%), osteolytic bone lesions, and/or an increasing tumor mass.

Amyloidosis accounts for about 4,000 deaths per year in the US. It usually has the same pathology as MGUS, except that the M Ig forms pathological deposits in various tissues – generally as the intact or fragmented Ig light chain [5].

Smoldering myeloma has a stable intramedullary tumor cell content of >10%, but no osteolytic lesions or other complications of malignant MM.

Progression of intramedullary myeloma is associated with increasingly severe secondary features (lytic bone lesions, anemia, immunodeficiency, and renal impairment), and, in a fraction of patients, the occurrence of tumors in extramedullary locations, including the peripheral blood. Extramedullary myeloma is a more aggressive tumor, which is often called primary or secondary plasma cell leukemia, depending on whether preceding intramedullary myeloma has been recognized.

Based on an analysis of 71 patients, the Durie–Salmon clinical staging system (see **Table 1**) was developed to correlate clinical features with an estimate of myeloma cell mass [6]. This was found to have prognostic value, and for the last 25 years has been the gold standard for the stratification of myeloma patients. More recently, the International Myeloma Working Group has correlated clinical features with survival in 11,171 cases and developed

	Stage I	Stage II	Stage III
Definition	All of the following	Neither Stage I nor Stage III	One or more of the following
Clinical features	Hemoglobin >10 g/dL Calcium <12 mg/dL ≤1 bone lesion Low M component: IgG <5 g/dL IgA <3 g/dL Bence Jones <4 g/dL		Hemoglobin <8.5 g/dL Calcium >12 mg/dL >3 bone lesions High M component: IgG >7 g/dL IgA >5 g/dL Bence Jones >12 g/dL
Myeloma cell concentration ($\times 10^{12}$ cells/m^2)	<0.6	0.6–1.2	>1.2
Subclassification (either A or B) A: Creatinine level <2.0 mg/dL B: Creatinine level ≥2.0 mg/dL			

Table 1. The Durie–Salmon Staging System [6]. M: monoclonal.

the International Staging System [7]. On univariate analysis (with hazard ratio), the important prognostic variables were a β_2-microglobulin concentration of ≥3.5 μg/mL (1.78), a creatinine concentration of ≥2 mg/dL (1.76), a platelet concentration of <130,000 cells/μL (1.71), an age of ≥65 years (1.63), a greater than normal lactate dehydrogenase concentration (1.52), a hemoglobin concentration of <10 g/dL (1.50), an albumin concentration of <3.5 g/dL (1.34), a ≥33% proportion of cells in the bone marrow that are plasma cells (1.34), and a C-reactive protein concentration of ≥0.8 mg/dL (1.30). Based on multivariate analysis, β_2-microglobulin and albumin were identified as independent prognostic factors, and three stages of approximately equal size were identified:

- Stage I (β_2-microglobulin concentration <3.5 μg/mL and albumin concentration ≥3.5 g/dL); median survival time = 62 months

- Stage II (β_2-microglobulin concentration <3.5 μg/mL and albumin concentration <3.5 g/dL, or β_2-microglobulin concentration 3.5–5.5 μg/mL); median survival time = 44 months

- Stage III (β_2-microglobulin concentration ≥5.5 μg/mL); median survival time = 29 months

Compared with the Durie–Salmon staging system, the International Staging System provides a more powerful discrimination between staging groups and a more even distribution of patients among stages. A newer classification system based on genetic abnormalities is currently being developed (see below).

MM is a tumor with a low rate of proliferation. The plasma cell labeling index, typically detecting <1% of tumor cells actively synthesizing DNA until late in the disease, is considered a better prognostic indicator than the tumor cell content in the bone marrow alone [8].

Epidemiology

Prevalence and incidence

MGUS

The prevalence (ie, the number of cases in a defined population at a certain time) of an M protein in people >25 years old was originally determined by paper electrophoresis in Varmland, Sweden, in 1965 [9]. Out of 6,995 consecutive serum samples tested, 0.9% (64 serum samples) contained an M protein. Only one subject had MM, and 63 cases were classified as MGUS, giving an MGUS prevalence of 901 per 100,000 people.

The incidence (ie, the number of new cases developing in a defined population over a defined period of time) of MGUS has not been determined. However, two registry studies have helped to provide a rough estimate: in the Netherlands, the incidence is estimated at 16 per 100,000 people [10], and in Iceland, 10 per 100,000 people [10,11].

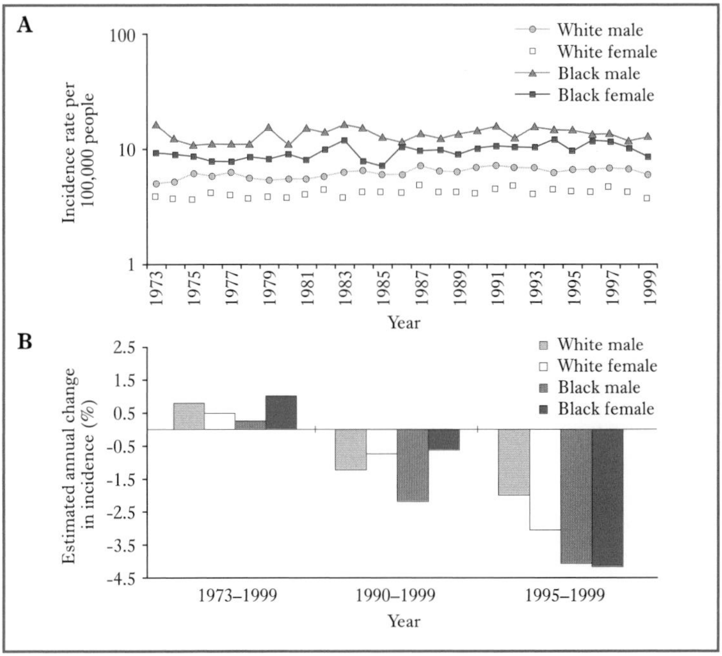

Figure 1. (A) Average annual age-specific incidence rates of multiple myeloma (MM) in the US, 1973–1999. **(B)** Estimated annual percentage change in these rates. Rates are age-adjusted to the 2000 US standard [1].

MM

The frequency with which MM is identified in a population is strongly influenced by age, race, and the availability of good medical care. In the US, the Surveillance, Epidemiology, and End Results (SEER) program has provided MM incidence data since 1973. For the 1995–1999 period, the average annual age-adjusted (2000 US standard) incidence rate per 100,000 people in the US was 5.6: 6.5 for white men, 4.2 for white women, 13.1 for black men, and 10.3 for black women (see **Figure 1**) [1]. The incidence of MM is slightly more common in men than women, and more than twice as common in blacks than whites. In many parts of the world, the incidence of MM appeared to increase markedly between 1950 and 1980. In the US, the incidence rate increased by 0.9% per year up until the early 1990s. This increase has now plateaued, and, over the last 10 years, the incidence rate in the US has possibly decreased slightly. The lifetime risk for being diagnosed with MM is 0.66% for men and 0.55% for women [1].

In 1999, about 47,709 people in the US were known to be living with MM: 18,530 white men, 20,618 white women, 4,066 black men, and 4,495 black women. This gives a prevalence of 17 per 100,000 people. It may seem surprising that, in the US, white women have the lowest incidence of MM but are currently the most prevalent subpopulation, and that black men have the highest incidence of MM and are the least prevalent subpopulation. This can be explained by the increased frequency of white women in the older US population, which is the age-group most at risk.

Age

During the period 1995–1999, in the US the median age of diagnosis of MM was 71 years, ranging from a median of 66 years in black men to a median of 73 years in white women [1]. MM was only rarely detected in patients under the age of 35 years (0.6% of all MM cases diagnosed during this period) [1]. The incidence progressively increases with age, reaching 40.3 per 100,000 people in the 80–84 years age-group [1]. The frequency of MGUS also increases with age. Axelsson et al. detected an M protein in 0.2% of subjects aged 30–49 years, 1.4% of subjects aged 50–69 years, and 4% of subjects aged 70–89 years [9]. Surveys of the serum electrophoresis patterns of nonagenarians have reported that 19% of these sera contain M proteins [12,13].

Race

The age-adjusted incidence (world standard population) of MM from worldwide, selected, population-based cancer registries ranges from 0.5 per 100,000 people in Hawaiian-Japanese males to 8.2 per 100,000 people in black males in the San Francisco/Oakland Bay area [14]. This suggests significant differences in the incidence of MM in different races. This view is supported by the observation that the incidence of MM – age-adjusted to the 1970 US standard – in Chinese males (2.3 per

100,000 people) and Japanese males (1.7 per 100,000 people) living in San Francisco/Oakland and Hawaii is distinctly lower than the incidence in white males (4.6 per 100,000 people) in the same regions [15]. The average annual age-adjusted (2000 US standard) incidence rates for US blacks (males: 13.1 per 100,000 people; females: 10.3 per 100,000 people) are more than double those for US whites [1]. The prevalence of MGUS is also more then twofold higher in blacks [16].

Etiology

The induction of plasma cell neoplasms is probably a multistep process. Genetic factors are likely to play a role in making a person susceptible to a change that results in the proliferation of a plasma cell precursor, thus forming a stable clone of plasma cells producing an M protein, as in MGUS. The conversion of the controlled, stable monoclone of MGUS into the uncontrolled, progressive, malignant tumor of MM probably requires one or more additional changes.

Radiation exposure

In 1979, an analysis of atomic bomb survivors in Japan identified an increased incidence of MM, which was apparent 20 years or more after exposure [17]. In 1994, an analysis employing dosimetry estimates in the same population, with 12 additional years of follow-up, did not confirm this [18]. Similarly, the frequency of MGUS does not appear to have increased in this cohort of patients [19]. In addition, studies have not confirmed an increased risk of MM among workers at nuclear power plants [20,21].

Socioeconomic status

Up until the early 1980s, MM was reported to cause increased mortality rates in members of the higher levels of society. This association was probably made because the disease was underascertained in the poor and uneducated. The reduced detection of MM in lower socioeconomic groups has gradually decreased with time. A case-control study done in 1984 at Duke University, NC, US, failed to demonstrate any association of MM with family income, education, occupation, dwelling size, or index of crowding in the home [22].

Environmental exposures

Riedel et al. reviewed 53 case-control, prospective, proportionate incidence/mortality studies that reported positive associations between specific occupations/industries and MM [14]. Employment in agriculture (predominantly farming) is the occupation most frequently associated with MM, and this association has been detected in most of the studies performed [23–25]. The reasons for the increased incidence are unclear although it has been postulated that it may relate to herbicides, farm animals or other environmental exposures. In addition, an increased incidence of MM has been noted in some, but not all, studies of workers employed in the industries of painting, metal work, rubber manufacturing, wood, leather and textiles, and petroleum production, as well as those exposed to asbestos, benzene, diesel exhaust, and hair dye.

Chronic antigen stimulation

Clinicians have long wondered whether chronic antigen stimulation plays a role in the pathogenesis of MM. It is hypothesized that a malignant transformation occurs in one of the responding cells during the proliferative immune response. There have been several attempts to correlate the occurrence of MM with a past history of exposure to viral or bacterial infections, immunizations, allergies, allergy desensitization therapy, and autoimmune diseases, but the results are inconsistent [23]. However, there appears to be an association between rheumatoid arthritis and MM, noted in several studies, and this is consistent with a role for chronic antigenic stimulation in the development of MM [26–29].

The discovery of an HIV-1 seropositive patient with MM, whose IgG/κ M protein specifically recognized the HIV-1 p24 gag antigen, suggests that the antigen-driven response to the viral infection played a role in the pathogenesis of MM in this patient [30]. In a prospective study of 239 patients with hepatitis C virus (HCV)-positive chronic liver disease and 98 with HCV-negative chronic liver disease, MGUS was detected in 11% of the HCV-positive, and only 1% of the HCV-negative patients [31].

Genetic factors

The following observations suggest that genetic factors play an important role in the pathogenesis of neoplasms:

- There are striking differences in the incidence of plasmacytomas in inbred strains of mice.
- There are racial differences in the incidence of plasma cell neoplasms.
- Familial MM occurs.

Murine plasma cell tumors

There are striking differences in the incidence of MGUS in different inbred strains of mice. About 60% of C57BL/Ka mice develop one or more M proteins (usually IgG) by the age of 24 months, while it is almost never seen in BALB/c and CBA/Rij mice [32]. In contrast, BALB/c mice are most susceptible to oil-induced plasmacytomas, while the C57BL/Ka strain is relatively resistant [33].

Racial differences in the incidence of MM and MGUS

There appear to be significant differences in the incidence of MM and MGUS among different races. The low incidence of MM in Japanese and Chinese populations is maintained when these populations move to the US (including Hawaii) [15]. This suggests that the incidence of disease in these populations is determined more by genetic than environmental factors.

Familial plasma cell neoplasia

Several families have been reported to have multiple family members with MM and MGUS (of the IgG, IgA, light chain, and IgD varieties) [34]. In the 41 families described, MM or MGUS was detected in seven first-degree relations (parent and child), was most frequent in 26 second-degree relatives (siblings), and was much less frequent in more distant relatives.

Pathophysiology

The development of overt MM is most likely to be a multistep process, which includes an ordered series of genetic changes that accumulate in the malignant plasma cell, the development of changes in the BM microenvironment that support tumor growth, and a failure of the immune system to control the disease.

Genomic instability

The karyotypic features of MM are more similar to those of epithelial tumors and the blast phase of chronic myelogenous leukemia than the karyotypic features of other hematopoietic tumors [35]. Numeric chromosomal abnormalities are present in virtually all MM tumors and most, if not all, MGUS tumors [4]. There is nonrandom involvement of various chromosomes in different MM tumors, and often heterogeneity among cells within a tumor.

Comparative genomic hybridization studies show that unbalanced chromosome structural changes are present in all plasma cell leukemias and most, if not all, MM tumors [36]. Chromosomal gains that recur in >30% of MM tumors are seen on 1q, 3q, 9q, 11q, and 15q – the consequences of which remain to be determined – and the most frequent site of chromosomal loss is on 13q.

A more comprehensive view of chromosomal abnormalities is provided by spectral karyotype analyses, though these are complicated by the fact that metaphase spreads can only be obtained in about 20% of cases [37]. It is thought that karyotypic complexity increases during tumor progression, though karyotypic progression has not been well documented. It is important to understand how the karyotype correlates with disease severity, because the detection of an abnormal karyotype correlates with an increased plasma cell labeling index and poor prognosis [8]. Hypodiploidy is associated with a poorer prognosis than hyperdiploidy [38].

Immunoglobulin gene translocations

Primary versus secondary translocations

Primary translocations are thought to occur early in pathogenesis, whereas secondary translocations are involved in progression [39]. During the pathogenesis of MM, most primary translocations are simple reciprocal translocations that juxtapose an oncogene and one of the Ig enhancers. They are mediated mainly by errors in Ig heavy-chain switch recombination, but are also sometimes caused by errors in somatic hypermutation during plasma cell generation in germinal centers [39]. Since all three B cell DNA modification mechanisms seem to be inactive in normal and tumor plasma cells, secondary translocations must be mediated by other mechanisms, such as those active in all forms of advanced tumors. The only definitive way to discern whether translocations are primary or secondary would be to document the time(s) at which they occur during the progression of individual tumors, which would be difficult and has not been done before.

Primary translocations involving an Ig locus

Translocations involving an Ig locus are present in most MM tumors [40]. Fluorescence *in situ* hybridization (FISH) analysis identifies Ig heavy-chain translocations by dissociation of probes that flank the 1 Mb Ig heavy-chain locus, enabling the analysis of interphase tumor cells. The incidence of heavy-chain translocations increases with the stage of tumorigenesis, from 50% in MGUS to 90% in human myeloma cell lines (HMCL) [39–42]. Light-chain translocations are less common: Igλ translocations are identified in approximately 10% of MGUS tumors and 20% of advanced MM and HMCL, whereas Igκ translocations are rare (WM Kuehl, R Fonseca, personal communication, 2001). Four partner chromosomes (4p16, 6p21, 11q13, and 16q23) and associated oncogenes that commonly become fused to Ig enhancers have the hallmarks of primary translocations, whereas additional infrequent but recurrent partner loci often have the characteristics of secondary translocations [39].

Despite the promiscuity of translocation partners, most Ig translocations involve just three groups of genes. The first group contains cyclins D1 (on 11q13), D3 (on 6p21), and possibly D2 (on 12p13). These are translocated in about 20%–25% of MM tumors [43,44].

The second group of genes is located on 4p16 and encodes two proteins: MMSET (a putative histone methyltransferase involved in chromatin remodeling) and fibroblast growth factor receptor 3 (FGFR3), an oncogenic receptor tyrosine kinase. These are translocated in about 15% of tumors. All of the breakpoints occur in a switch region, resulting in the simultaneous dysregulation of *FGFR3* from der(14) (the translocation derivative that contains the centromere of chromosome 14) and *MMSET* from der(4) [45,46].

Unlike *FGFR3*, *MMSET* is not a well-characterized oncogene, but the lack of variant translocations, and the fact that loss of der(4) has never been observed in MM, indicate that dysregulation of *MMSET* is important for malignant transformation. This hypothesis is supported by the fact that *MMSET* is homologous to *MLL*, which is involved in 11q23 translocations in acute leukemia [47].

The third group of genes commonly involved in Ig gene translocations comprises the code for two b-zip transcription factors – c-Maf (encoded on 16q23) and MAFB (encoded on 20q11). These are translocated in about 10% of tumors [48,49] (PL Bergsagel, WM Kuehl, J Shaughnessy, unpublished data). The centromeric t(14;16) 16q23 breakpoints occur within the introns of a very large gene, *WWOX*, that spans a fragile site (FRA16D). These breakpoints are located up to 1 Mb centromeric from c-*maf*. Despite an apparent similarity of function with *c-maf*,

MafB translocations have structural features that indicate that they are secondary and not primary translocations (PL Bergsagel, WM Kuehl, unpublished data).

It is clear that these translocations identify distinct subtypes of MM with important prognostic implications. A follow-up study from the Intergroupe Francophone du Myelome using interphase FISH analysis to detect Ig heavy-chain gene translocations found that 13% of patients with t(4;14) had a poor overall survival rate (23% at 80 months), and did not appear to achieve lasting disease control with high-dose chemotherapy [50]. In contrast, 16% of patients with t(11;14) translocations had an especially good prognosis with this therapy (88% survival at 80 months). Survival in both of these subgroups was independent of chromosomal deletions on 13q.

Similar results have also been noted for patients treated with conventional chemotherapy [51]. The presence of translocations t(4;14) (26 vs 45 months; $P < 0.001$) and t(14;16) (16 vs 41 months; $P = 0.003$), as well as deletions at 17p13 (23 vs 44 months; $P = 0.005$) and 13q14 (35 vs 51 months; $P = 0.028$), were associated with shorter survival times. Although the t(11;14) translocation was associated with a slightly longer survival time (50 vs 39 months; $P = 0.332$), the difference was much smaller than was noted among the French patients treated with high-dose chemotherapy, and did not reach statistical significance. These provocative data suggest that patients with the t(11;14) translocation may especially benefit from high-dose chemotherapy.

Secondary translocations dysregulate myc

Dysregulation of *myc* occurs in several B cell tumors. Despite many prior efforts to identify translocations that juxtapose c-*myc* and Ig sequences in MM, this was thought to be a rare event until advanced cytogenetic methods became available. In MM, complex translocations dysregulate c-*myc* as a late progression event that is associated with enhanced cell proliferation. Three-color FISH analyses of metaphase chromosomes show that 88% of HMCL and 45% of advanced primary MM tumors have karyotypic abnormalities involving *myc* [52].

Most of the karyotypic abnormalities involving *myc* are complex translocations and insertions that are often nonreciprocal, and frequently involve three different chromosomes. The karyotypic abnormalities often, but not always, juxtapose c-*myc* and an Ig enhancer. Interphase FISH analyses indicate that c-*myc* is rearranged in 15% of MM tumors across all stages; it is more frequent in the advanced stages, and is often heterogeneous among cells within the tumor [53]. These results support a model for MM in which dysregulation of *myc* occurs as a very late progression event mediated by secondary translocations that do not involve B cell-specific DNA modification mechanisms [39].

A tumor suppressor gene on chromosome 13?

Monoallelic loss of 13q sequences is one of the most frequent abnormalities in MM (approx. 50% of untreated cases identified by interphase FISH analyses), and is an independent predictor of a poor prognosis [54]. Most often there is chromosome 13 monosomy, with selective loss of 13q sequences by interstitial deletion or translocation occurring much less frequently. The minimum region of deletion appears to be at 13q14, but biallelic deletion is rare. Notably, trisomy of chromosome 13 is also rare. The frequency of chromosome 13q loss increases with disease stage, from 20% of patients with MGUS to nearly 70% in plasma cell leukemia or HMCL [54].

In most patients with MGUS, only a subset of tumor cells has the 13q abnormality; in MM patients with this abnormality, it is found in virtually all tumor cells. These results indicate that chromosome 13 losses begin in MGUS and increase in MM. However, the nearly uniform presence of this abnormality in MGUS and MM tumors with t(4;14) raises the possibility that this abnormality might occur as a very early event in tumors with this translocation [55].

Studies of other types of tumors show that both copies of the retinoblastoma (*RB*) gene at 13q14 must be inactivated to eliminate its tumor suppressor function [56]. However, biallelic deletion, inactivating mutations, and lack of *RB* expression appear to occur only rarely, even in advanced MM tumors and cell lines. This suggests that another tumor suppressor gene may be involved in the pathogenesis of MM. In addition, there is evidence that a number of other well-known tumor suppressor genes – *p16*, *p18*, *PTEN*, and *p53* – are sometimes involved in the progression of MM [57–61].

Activating mutations of ras and FGFR3

Activating mutations of N-*ras* or K-*ras* oncogenes distinguish MM from MGUS. In one large study, activating mutations of *ras* at codons 12, 13, or 61 were identified in approximately 40% of MM tumors at the time of diagnosis, with a limited analysis indicating mutations in 49% of tumors at the time of relapse; 60% of the mutations were in N-*ras*, and 40% in K-*ras* [62]. The frequency of activating *ras* mutations is relatively independent of the plasma cell labeling index and stage of MM. The same mutations are found in 45% of HMCL patients [63]. However, <5% of MGUS tumors have *ras* mutations (T Rasmussen, personal communication, 2002). Tumors that overexpress *FGFR3* as a result of a t(4;14) translocation can have activating mutations of *ras* or *FGFR3* but not both. This is consistent with constitutive activation of the mitogen-activated protein kinase (MAPK) pathway downstream of both *FGFR3* and *ras*, and suggests that it may be redundant to activate both pathways [63]. Transfection studies of interleukin (IL)-6-dependent HMCL show that activating mutations of either N-*ras*/K-*ras* or *FGFR3* enhance growth and decrease the amount of IL-6 that is required for tumor survival and growth (see below) [64].

IL-6 and IGF-1

Interaction of IL-6 with its receptor (IL-6r) – present on normal plasmablasts and MGUS or MM tumor cells – usually results in enhanced cell survival and growth [65]. In many *in vivo* or *in vitro* primary MM tumors, as well as IL-6-dependent HMCL or normal plasmablasts *in vitro*, antibodies against IL-6 increase apoptosis and decrease growth. This suggests that IL-6 is a critical paracrine factor usually involved in the early pathogenesis of MM, though IL-6 independence can occur during disease progression.

There is increasing evidence to suggest that insulin-like growth factor (IGF)-1 is another paracrine factor that enhances tumor survival and growth [66]. Both cytokines are thought to increase proliferation by activating the *ras*–MAPK pathway. Enhanced survival is mediated by different pathways: IL-6 activates a transcription factor, STAT3, which increases the expression of antiapoptotic genes, including *mcl*-1, $bclX_L$, and *pim*-1, as well as c-*myc*, which presumably enhances cell proliferation [67,68]. STAT3 also seems to activate the phosphatidylinositol (PI)3-kinase–Akt pathway [69]. IGF-1 also activates PI3-kinase, which phosphorylates BAD and Akt to inhibit apoptosis [66]. Mutations in the *ras* (MAPK pathway) or *FGFR3* (MAPK and STAT3 pathways) enhance survival and proliferation, but do not always result in IL-6 independence.

The bone marrow microenvironment

The pathogenesis of most tumors includes complex and evolving mutual interactions that affect the number and phenotype of both the tumor cells and a variety of normal BM stromal cells (BMSCs) [70]. Normal, long-lived plasma cells and all stages of intramedullary tumor are dependent on the BM microenvironment for survival, growth, and differentiation [71]. This microenvironment includes the extracellular matrix and five kinds of BMSCs: fibroblastic stromal cells, osteoblasts, osteoclasts, vascular endothelial cells, and lymphocytes. For intramedullary MM, there are a number of biological phenomena that are affected by these tumor–host interactions:

- homing of the tumor to the BM

- spread of the tumor via the bloodstream from one site to a second site within the BM
- generation of paracrine factors that are involved in the survival, differentiation, and proliferation of tumor cells
- angiogenesis
- osteoclastogenesis and osteolysis
- inhibition of osteogenesis
- humoral and cellular immunodeficiency
- anemia

The most important of these phenomena are now discussed in greater detail.

Homing

Homing seems to involve selective adhesion of MM cells to BM endothelial cells, transendothelial migration, and MM cell adhesion to BMSCs – a process that involves stromal-derived factor 1 and IGF-1 as potential chemoattractants secreted by BM endothelial cells and BMSCs [72–74].

Paracrine factors

In the presence of normal and tumor plasma cells, these paracrine cells and the various normal BMSCs secrete cytokines (IL-6, IGF-1, IL-1β, transforming growth factor-β, and tumor necrosis factor [TNF]-α) as a result of mutual interactions mediated by direct cell–cell contact, cell–matrix contact, or other secreted factors [75–80]. For example, HMCL and MM tumor cells secrete vascular endothelial growth factor (VEGF), which not only stimulates BMSCs to secrete increased levels of IL-6 to enhance the growth and survival of MM tumor cells, but also increases the expression and secretion of VEGF from the tumor cells [78].

Angiogenesis

Angiogenesis is correlated with disease activity – there is a low level of angiogenesis in primary amyloidosis and MGUS, a somewhat higher level in smoldering myeloma, and markedly higher levels in active MM. The extent of angiogenesis is directly correlated with the plasma cell labeling index and inversely correlated with the length of patient survival. Secreted VEGF from MM cells is thought to interact with receptors on endothelial cells to enhance their migration and proliferation. Additional factors (eg, basic fibroblast growth factor) generated by MM tumor cells or other BM cells might also enhance angiogenesis. Nonetheless, the precise role of angiogenesis in MM remains to be established [81,82].

Osteolysis

Osteolysis, which occurs predominantly at the interface of bone and MM (but not MGUS), is mediated by increased osteoclast activity and decreased osteoblast activity at these sites [83]. The mechanism causing decreased osteoblast activity is unclear, but many potential osteoclast-activating factors (IL-6, IL-1β, parathyroid hormone-related protein, hepatocyte growth factor, and TNF-α) are generated by the interactions of tumor and BM cells.

Two mechanisms of osteoclast activation are particularly notable. The first involves macrophage inflammatory protein-1α, which is secreted by MM cells and functions as an osteoclast chemotactic and maturation factor [84,85]. The second mechanism involves a receptor called receptor activator of nuclear factor-κB (RANK), which binds the cytokine RANK ligand (RANKL). This pathway appears to be the key regulator of osteoclastogenesis. RANKL, which is normally expressed as a membrane-bound ligand on osteoblasts and T cells, interacts with RANK on an osteoclast precursor to generate an active osteoclast [86,87]. Normal megakaryocytes and BMSCs secrete a "decoy receptor" called osteoprotegerin (OPG), which competes with RANK for RANKL. The direct interaction of α4β1-integrin on MM tumor cells with vascular cell adhesion molecule-1 on BMSCs causes a marked

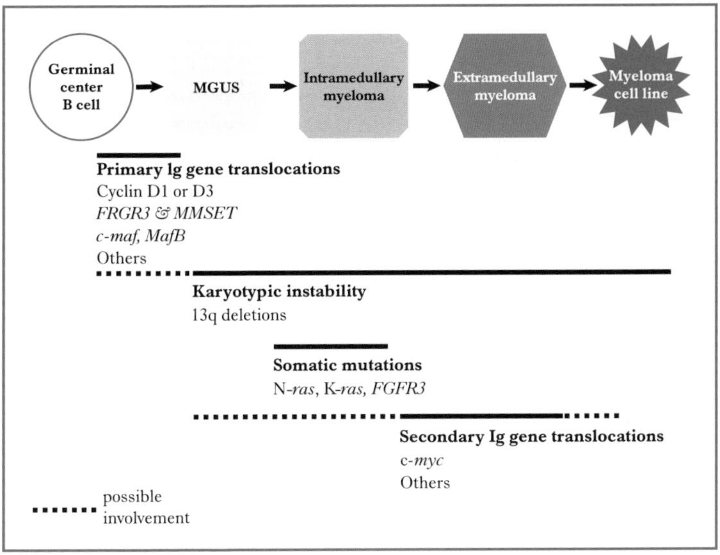

Figure 2. Multistep molecular pathogenesis of multiple myeloma (MM). A minimum number of intermediates in the MM pathogenesis pathway are depicted. Horizontal lines indicate the approximate timing of specific oncogenic events, with solid lines indicating the most likely time that these events will occur. MGUS: monoclonal gammopathy of undetermined significance.

decrease in OPG secretion as well as enhanced expression of RANKL by stromal cells, and perhaps also by tumor cells.

Summary

The combined clinical, pathologic, genetic, and phenotypic observations discussed in this chapter suggest a working model of MM progression (see **Figure 2**). It is postulated that there is an immortalizing event in the germinal center – most frequently a primary Ig heavy-chain translocation occurring at the time of switch recombination and somatic hypermutation, though a substantial fraction of tumors have no Ig translocation. Some tumors without a primary Ig translocation may have activated oncogenes or inactivated tumor suppressor genes as a result of a spillover of Ig heavy-chain switch recombination or somatic hypermutation to non-Ig loci.

A primary Ig translocation results in the ectopic expression of an oncogene (cyclin D1, cyclin D3, *FGFR3/MMSET*, c-*maf*, or *mafB*) that causes proliferation of the long-lived plasmablast/plasma cell. Marked karyotypic abnormalities are already present in premalignant MGUS, perhaps as a consequence of telomeric crisis. However, since the temporal relation between karyotypic abnormalities and Ig heavy-chain translocations is not understood, it is possible that karyotypic instability is the initiating oncogenic event in MM, whether or not an Ig heavy-chain translocation is present. Secondary translocations contribute to subsequent disease progression.

In MGUS and MM, the role of a possible tumor suppressor gene on 13q remains enigmatic. However, progression from MGUS to MM is associated with activating mutations of *ras* or *FGFR3*. This progression seems to flip a molecular switch that results in osteolytic bone lesions mediated by osteoclastogenesis, angiogenesis, and enhanced growth of the MM clone. Further tumor progression, and especially extramedullary growth, is associated with increased proliferation (increased DNA labeling index), mutations of *p53*, and secondary translocations that dysregulate c-*myc*.

References

1. Ries LAG, Eisner MP, Kosary CL et al, editors. *SEER Cancer Statistics Review, 1973–1999*. Bethesda, MD: National Cancer Institute, 2002. Available from: URL: http://seer.cancer.gov/csr/1973_1999. Accessed on June 3, 2003.
2. Lynch HT, Sanger WG, Pirruccello S et al. Familial multiple myeloma: a family study and review of the literature. *J Natl Cancer Inst* 2001;93:1479–83.
3. Kyle RA, Therneau TM, Rajkumar SV et al. A long-term study of prognosis in monoclonal gammopathy of undetermined significance. *N Engl J Med* 2002;346:564–9.
4. Avet-Loiseau H, Facon T, Daviet A et al. 14q32 translocations and monosomy 13 observed in monoclonal gammopathy of undetermined significance delineate a multistep process for the oncogenesis of multiple myeloma. Intergroupe Francophone du Myelome. *Cancer Res* 1999;59:4546–50.
5. Hayman SR, Bailey RJ, Jalal SM et al. Translocations involving the immunoglobulin heavy-chain locus are possible early genetic events in patients with primary systemic amyloidosis. *Blood* 2001;98:2266–8.

6. Durie BG, Salmon SE. A clinical staging system for multiple myeloma. Correlation of measured myeloma cell mass with presenting clinical features, response to treatment, and survival. *Cancer* 1975;36:842–54.
7. Greipp PR, San Miguel JF, Durie BG et al. A new international staging system (ISS) for multiple myeloma (MM) from the International Myeloma Working Group. *Blood* 2003;102:644a (Abstr.).
8. Rajkumar SV, Fonseca R, Dewald GW et al. Cytogenetic abnormalities correlate with the plasma cell labeling index and extent of bone marrow involvement in myeloma. *Cancer Genet Cytogenet* 1999;113:73–7.
9. Axelsson U, Bachmann R, Hallen J. Frequency of pathological proteins (M-components) in 6,995 sera from an adult population. *Acta Med Scand* 1966;179:235–47.
10. Ong F, Hermans J, Noordijk EM et al. A population-based registry on paraproteinaemia in The Netherlands. Comprehensive Cancer Centre West, Leiden, The Netherlands. *Br J Haematol* 1997;99:914–20.
11 Ogmundsdottir HM, Haraldsdottir V, M Johannesson G et al. Monoclonal gammopathy in Iceland: a population-based registry and follow-up. *Br J Haematol* 2002;118:166–73.
12. Englisova M, Englis M, Kyral V et al. Changes of immunoglobulin synthesis in old people. *Exp Gerontol* 1968;3:125–7.
13. Radl J, Sepers JM, Skvaril F et al. Immunoglobulin patterns in humans over 95 years of age. *Clin Exp Immunol* 1975;22:84–90.
14. Riedel DA, Pottern LM, Blattner WA. Epidemiology of multiple myeloma. In: Wiernik PH, Canellos GP, Kyle RA et al, editors. *Neoplastic Diseases of the Blood*. 2nd edition. New York, NY: Churchill Livingstone, 1991:347–72.
15. Devesa SS. Descriptive epidemiology of multiple myeloma. In: Obrams GI, Potter M, editors. *Epidemiology and Biology of Multiple Myeloma*. Berlin: Springer Verlag, 1991:3–12.
16. Cohen HJ, Crawford J, Rao MK et al. Racial differences in the prevalence of monoclonal gammopathy in a community-based sample of the elderly. *Am J Med* 1998;104:439–44.
17. Ichimaru M, Ishimaru T, Mikami M et al. Multiple myeloma among atomic bomb survivors in Hiroshima and Nagasaki, 1950–76: relationship to radiation dose absorbed by marrow. *J Natl Cancer Inst* 1982;69:323–8.
18. Preston DL, Kusumi S, Tomonaga M et al. Cancer incidence in atomic bomb survivors. Part III. Leukemia, lymphoma and multiple myeloma, 1950–1987. *Radiat Res* 1994;137(2 Suppl.):68S-97S.
19. Neriishi K, Yoshimoto Y, Carter RL et al. Monoclonal gammopathy in atomic bomb survivors. *Radiat Res* 1993;133:351–9.
20. Muirhead CR, Goodill AA, Haylock RG et al. Occupational radiation exposure and mortality: second analysis of the National Registry for Radiation Workers. *J Radiol Prot* 1999;19:3–26.
21. Wing S, Richardson D, Wolf S et al. A case control study of multiple myeloma at four nuclear facilities. *Ann Epidemiol* 2000;10:144–53.
22. Johnston JM, Grufferman S, Bourguet CC et al. Socioeconomic status and risk of multiple myeloma. *J Epidemiol Community Health* 1985;39:175–8.
23. Riedel DA, Pottern LM. The epidemiology of multiple myeloma. *Hematol Oncol Clin North Am* 1992;6:225–47.
24. Pukkala E, Notkola V. Cancer incidence among Finnish farmers, 1979–93. *Cancer Causes Control* 1997;8:25–33.
25. Kristensen P, Andersen A, Irgens LM et al. Incidence and risk factors of cancer among men and women in Norwegian agriculture. *Scand J Work Environ Health* 1996;22:14–26.
26. Eriksson M. Rheumatoid arthritis as a risk factor for multiple myeloma: a case-control study. *Eur J Cancer* 1993;29A:259–63.

27. Katusic S, Beard CM, Kurland LT et al. Occurrence of malignant neoplasms in the Rochester, Minnesota, rheumatoid arthritis cohort. *Am J Med* 1985;78:50–5.
28. Isomaki HA, Hakulinen T, Joutsenlahti U. Excess risk of lymphomas, leukemia and myeloma in patients with rheumatoid arthritis. *J Chronic Dis* 1978;31:691–6.
29. Hakulinen T, Isomaki H, Knekt P. Rheumatoid arthritis and cancer studies based on linking nationwide registries in Finland. *Am J Med* 1985;78:29–32.
30. Konrad RJ, Kricka LJ, Goodman DB et al. Brief report: myeloma-associated paraprotein directed against the HIV-1 p24 antigen in an HIV-1-seropositive patient. *N Engl J Med* 1993;328:1817–9.
31. Andreone P, Zignego AL, Cursaro C et al. Prevalence of monoclonal gammopathies in patients with hepatitis C virus infection. *Ann Intern Med* 1998;129:294–8.
32. Radl J, Hollander CF, van den Berg P et al. Idiopathic paraproteinaemia. I. Studies in an animal model – the ageing C57BL/KaLwRij mouse. *Clin Exp Immunol* 1978;33:395–402.
33. Potter M, Pumphrey JG, Bailey DW. Genetics of susceptibility to plasmacytoma induction. I. BALB/cAnN (C), C57BL/6N (B6), C57BL/Ka (BK), (C times B6)F1, (C times BK)F1, and C times B recombinant-inbred strains. *J Natl Cancer Inst* 1975;54:1413–7.
34. Loth TS, Perrotta AL, Lima J et al. Genetic aspects of familial multiple myeloma. *Mil Med* 1991;156:430–3.
35. Mitelman Database of Chromosome Aberrations in Cancer (2003). Mitelman F, Johansson B, Mertens F, editors. Available from: URL: http://cgap.nci.nih.gov/Chromosomes/Mitelman
36. Gutierrez NC, Hernandez JM, Garcia JL et al. Differences in genetic changes between multiple myeloma and plasma cell leukemia demonstrated by comparative genomic hybridization. *Leukemia* 2001;15:840–5.
37. Sawyer JR, Lukacs JL, Thomas EL et al. Multicolour spectral karyotyping identifies new translocations and a recurring pathway for chromosome loss in multiple myeloma. *Br J Haematol* 2001;112:167–74.
38. Smadja NV, Bastard C, Brigaudeau C et al. Hypodiploidy is a major prognostic factor in multiple myeloma. *Blood* 2001;98:2229–38.
39. Bergsagel PL, Kuehl WM. Chromosome translocations in multiple myeloma. *Oncogene* 2001;20:5611–22.
40. Bergsagel PL, Chesi MC, Nardini E et al. Promiscuous translocations into immunoglobulin heavy chain switch regions in multiple myeloma. *Proc Natl Acad Sci USA* 1996;93:13931–6.
41. Avet-Louseau H, Daviet A, Sauner S et al. Chromosome 13 abnormalities in multiple myeloma are mostly monosomy 13. *Br J Haematol* 2000;111:1116–7.
42. Avet-Louseau H. Nonrandom distribution of chromosomal abnormalities and correlation with clinical stage and prognostic presentation: a novel model for oncogenesis in multiple myeloma. *Program and abstracts of the VIII International Myeloma Workshop*, Banff, Alta., Canada, 4–8 May, 2001 (Abstr. S5).
43. Chesi M, Bergsagel PL, Brents LA et al. Dysregulation of cyclin D1 by translocation into an IgH gamma switch region in two multiple myeloma cell lines. *Blood* 1996;88:674–81.
44. Shaughnessy J, Gabrea A, Qi Y et al. Cyclin D3 at 6p21 is dysregulated by recurrent chromosomal translocations to immunoglobulin loci in multiple myeloma. *Blood* 2001;98:217–23.
45. Chesi M, Nardini E, Brents LA et al. Frequent translocation t(4;14)(p16.3;q32.3) in multiple myeloma is associated with increased expression and activating mutations of fibroblast growth factor receptor 3. *Nat Genet* 1997;16:260–4.
46. Chesi M, Nardini E, Lim RS et al. The t(4;14) translocation in myeloma dysregulates both FGFR3 and a novel gene, MMSET, resulting in IgH/MMSET hybrid transcripts. *Blood* 1998;92:3025–34.

47. Ayton PM, Cleary ML. Molecular mechanisms of leukemogenesis mediated by MLL fusion proteins. *Oncogene* 2001;20:5695–707.
48. Chesi M, Bergsagel PL, Shonukan OO et al. Frequent dysregulation of the c-*maf* proto-oncogene at 16q23 by translocation to an Ig locus in multiple myeloma. *Blood* 1998;91:4457–63.
49. Hanamura I, Iida S, Akano Y et al. Ectopic expression of MAFB gene in human myeloma cells carrying (14;20)(q32;q11) chromosomal translocations. *Jpn J Cancer Res* 2001;92:638–44.
50. Moreau P, Facon T, Leleu X et al. Recurrent 14q32 translocations determine the prognosis of multiple myeloma, especially in patients receiving intensive chemotherapy. *Blood* 2002;100:1579–83.
51. Fonseca R., Blood E, Rue M et al. Clinical and biologic implications of recurrent genomic aberrations in myeloma. *Blood* 2003;101:4569–75.
52. Shou Y, Martelli ML, Gabrea A et al. Diverse karyotypic abnormalities of the c-*myc* locus associated with c-*myc* dysregulation and tumor progression in multiple myeloma. *Proc Natl Acad Sci USA* 2000;97:228–33.
53. Avet-Loiseau H, Gerson F, Magrangeas F et al. Rearrangements of the c-*myc* oncogene are present in 15% of primary human multiple myeloma tumors. *Blood* 2001;98:3082–6.
54. Zojer N, Konigsberg R, Ackermann J et al. Deletion of 13q14 remains an independent adverse prognostic variable in multiple myeloma despite its frequent detection by interphase fluorescence *in situ* hybridization. *Blood* 2000;95:1925–30.
55. Fonesca R, Oken MM, Greipp PR. The t(4;14)(p16.3;q32) is strongly associated with chromosome 13 abnormalities in both multiple myeloma and monoclonal gammopathy of undetermined significance. *Blood* 2001;98:1271–2.
56 Juge-Morineau N, Harousseau JL, Amiot M et al. The retinoblastoma susceptibility gene RB-1 in multiple myeloma. *Leuk Lymphoma* 1997;24:229–37.
57. Guillerm G, Gyan E, Wolowiec D et al. p16(INK4a) and p15(INK4b) gene methylations in plasma cells from monoclonal gammopathy of undetermined significance. *Blood* 2001;98:244–6.
58. Kulkarni MS, Daggett JL, Bender TP et al. Frequent inactivation of the cyclin-dependent kinase inhibitor p18 by homozygous deletion in multiple myeloma cell lines: ectopic p18 expression inhibits growth and induces apoptosis. *Leukemia* 2002;16:127–34.
59. Urashima M, Teoh G, Ogata A et al. Characterization of p16(INK4A) expression in multiple myeloma and plasma cell leukemia. *Clin Cancer Res* 1997;3:2173–9.
60. Neri A, Baldini L, Trecca D et al. p53 gene mutations in multiple myeloma are associated with advanced forms of malignancy. *Blood* 1993;81:128–35.
61. Ge NL, Rudikoff S. Expression of PTEN in PTEN-deficient multiple myeloma cells abolishes tumor growth *in vivo*. *Oncogene* 2000;19:4091–5.
62. Liu P, Leong T, Quam L et al. Activating mutations of N- and K-*ras* in multiple myeloma show different clinical associations: analysis of the Eastern Cooperative Oncology Group Phase III Trial. *Blood* 1996;88:2699–706.
63. Chesi M, Brents LA, Ely SA et al. Activated fibroblast growth factor receptor 3 is an oncogene that contributes to tumor progression in multiple myeloma. *Blood* 2001;97:729–36.
64. Billadeau D, Liu P, Jelinek D et al. Activating mutations in the N- and K-*ras* oncogenes differentially affect the growth properties of the IL-6-dependent myeloma cell line ANBL6. *Cancer Res* 1997;57:2268–75.
65. Klein B, Zhang XG, Lu ZY et al. Interleukin-6 in human multiple myeloma. *Blood* 1995;85:863–72.
66. Ge NL, Rudikoff S. Insulin-like growth factor I is a dual effector of multiple myeloma cell growth. *Blood* 2000;96:2856–61.

67. Catlett-Falcone R, Landowski TH, Oshiro MM et al. Constitutive activation of STAT3 signaling confers resistance to apoptosis in human U266 myeloma cells. *Immunity* 1999;10:105–15.
68. Puthier D, Derenne S, Barille S et al. Mcl-1 and Bcl-xL are co-regulated by IL-6 in human myeloma cells. *Br J Haematol* 1999;107:392–5.
69. Hideshima T, Nakamura N, Chauhan D et al. Biologic sequelae of interleukin-6 induced PI3-K/Akt signaling in multiple myeloma. *Oncogene* 2001;20:5991–6000.
70. Liotta LA, Kohn EC. The microenvironment of the tumour-host interface. *Nature* 2001;411:375–9.
71. Shain KH, Landowski TH, Dalton WS. The tumor microenvironment as a determinant of cancer cell survival: a possible mechanism for *de novo* drug resistance. *Curr Opin Oncol* 2000;12:557–63.
72. Asosingh K, Gunthert U, Bakkus MH et al. *In vivo* induction of insulin-like growth factor-I receptor and CD44v6 confers homing and adhesion to murine multiple myeloma cells. *Cancer Res* 2000;60:3096–104.
73. Asosingh K, Gunthert U, De Raeve H et al. A unique pathway in the homing of murine multiple myeloma cells: CD44v10 mediates binding to bone marrow endothelium. *Cancer Res* 2001;61:2862–5.
74. Van Riet I. Homing mechanisms of myeloma cells. *Pathol Biol (Paris)* 1999;47:98–108.
75. Cook G, Dumbar M, Franklin IM. The role of adhesion molecules in multiple myeloma. *Acta Haematol* 1997;97:81–9.
76. Costes V, Portier M, Lu ZY et al. Interleukin-1 in multiple myeloma: producer cells and their role in the control of IL-6 production. *Br J Haematol* 1998;103:1152–60.
77. Dankbar B, Padro T, Leo R et al. Vascular endothelial growth factor and interleukin-6 in paracrine tumor-stromal cell interactions in multiple myeloma. *Blood* 2000;95:2630–6.
78. Lokhorst HM, Lamme T, de Smet M et al. Primary tumor cells of myeloma patients induce interleukin-6 secretion in long-term bone marrow cultures. *Blood* 1994;84:2269–77.
79. Lacy MQ, Donovan KA, Heimbach JK et al. Comparison of interleukin-1β expression by *in situ* hybridization in monoclonal gammopathy of undetermined significance and multiple myeloma. *Blood* 1999;93:300–5.
80. Uchiyama H, Barut BA, Mohrbacher AF et al. Adhesion of human myeloma-derived cell lines to bone marrow stromal cells stimulates interleukin-6 secretion. *Blood* 1993;82:3712–20.
81. Rajkumar SV, Leong T, Roche PC et al. Prognostic value of bone marrow angiogenesis in multiple myeloma. *Clin Cancer Res* 2000;6:3111–6.
82. Vacca A, Ribatti D, Presta M et al. Bone marrow neovascularization, plasma cell angiogenic potential, and matrix metalloproteinase-2 secretion parallel progression of human multiple myeloma. *Blood* 1999;93:3064–73.
83. Roodman GD. Biology of osteoclast activation in cancer. *J Clin Oncol* 2001;19:3562–71.
84. Callander NS, Roodman GD. Myeloma bone disease. *Semin Hematol* 2001;38:276–85.
85. Han JH, Choi SJ, Kurihara N et al. Macrophage inflammatory protein-1α is an osteoclastogenic factor in myeloma that is independent of receptor activator of nuclear factor κB ligand. *Blood* 2001;97:3349–53.
86. Michigami T, Shimizu N, Williams PJ et al. Cell-cell contact between marrow stromal cells and myeloma cells via VCAM-1 and α(4)β(1)-integrin enhances production of osteoclast- stimulating activity. *Blood* 2000;96:1953–60.
87. Pearse RN, Sordillo EM, Yaccoby S et al. Multiple myeloma disrupts the TRANCE/osteoprotegerin cytokine axis to trigger bone destruction and promote tumor progression. *Proc Natl Acad Sci USA* 2001;98:11581–6.

2

Mechanisms of drug resistance and therapeutic implications

Kenneth H Shain & Melissa Alsina

Introduction

Despite recent advances in treatment, multiple myeloma (MM) remains an incurable disease, largely due to the emergence of drug resistance [1]. This resistance is characterized by a concomitant insensitivity to the drugs used in therapy, as well as to other unrelated cytotoxic agents – a phenomenon known as acquired multidrug resistance (MDR) [2–5].

Whilst acquired MDR has been shown to develop following chemotherapy, a number of reports have demonstrated that environmental factors may also modulate cellular sensitivity to multiple cytotoxic agents prior to chemotherapy, thus providing *de novo* MDR [6–11]. *De novo* MDR is of particular importance in MM due to the unique bone marrow (BM) dissemination of the disease.

It has been hypothesized that the microenvironment of BM may provide a sanctuary to MM cells. Through a network of survival factors – comprised of both soluble molecules and direct contact between tumor cells and their environment – the microenvironment favors the preferential homing of MM cells to the BM, along with drug resistance.

The clinical manifestation of MDR, whether acquired or *de novo*, is thought to be a major factor in treatment failure in MM and many other cancers. The ubiquitous nature of MDR has led to a large investigative effort into the identification of the cellular mechanisms involved in drug resistance. It is an effort that is spurred on by the principle that identifying these cellular determinants would facilitate the development of therapies to circumvent resistance. This chapter divides these findings into two general categories:

- acquired MDR
- *de novo* MDR, or MDR conferred by the microenvironment of the tumor

The mechanisms of both acquired and *de novo* MDR, and how an understanding of these mechanisms has impacted current and future treatment of MM, are discussed.

Acquired MDR

In MM, overall clinical success has been unachievable due to the expansion of MM cells that are refractory to therapy. One mechanism by which cancer cells become refractory involves the acquisition of mechanisms of resistance in the face of cytotoxic insult: cancer cells undergo molecular changes that facilitate an adaptation to the cytotoxic environment created by therapy. This selective process results in the acquisition of mechanisms that confer resistance to multiple classes of therapeutic agents – acquired MDR.

Much of what is known about the mechanisms of acquired MDR has been elucidated using *in vitro* systems that focus on cellular and molecular changes within individual cells selected under prolonged exposure to cytotoxic insult. The mechanisms of acquired MDR in MM can be divided into three subcategories (see **Table 1**):

- reduction of intracellular drug accumulation at target cells
- alteration of drug target
- antiapoptosis

	Mechanism of acquired multidrug resistance		
	Reduction of intracellular drug accumulation at target	**Alteration in drug target**	**Antiapoptotic factors**
Examples	Increased intracellular levels of P-glycoprotein	Reduced topoisomerase II expression	Increased levels of Bcl-2 protein family members
	Increased intracellular levels of multidrug resistance protein	Decreased levels of GR expression	Decreased levels of CD95 expression[1]
	Increased intracellular levels of breast cancer resistance protein	Deletion of GR hormone-binding domain	
	Increased intracellular levels of lung resistance protein/major vault protein		
	Drug detoxification		
	Decreased CD98 expression		

Table 1. Mechanisms of acquired multidrug resistance identified in multiple myeloma. GR: glucocorticoid receptor.
[1]Antiapoptotic. However, no direct link to drug resistance has been established.

Although these mechanisms of acquired MDR have been categorized, substantial evidence indicates that, within a given cell, MDR is multifactorial and often employs one or more of these subcategories of drug resistance [12,13].

Reduced intracellular drug accumulation at target cells

More than 20 years ago, reports demonstrated a correlation between acquired MDR following *in vitro* anthracycline selection and increased expression of the drug efflux pump P-glycoprotein (P-gp/MDR1) [2,3,14]. In MM cell lines, selection with doxorubicin correlated with decreased intracellular drug concentration, increased drug efflux, and overexpression of P-gp [2]. Consistent with the MDR phenotype, selection with doxorubicin resulted in resistance to mitoxantrone, acromycin, etoposide, and vincristine.

Subsequent studies demonstrated that other drug transporters, including multidrug resistance protein (MRP)1 and breast cancer resistance protein, are similarly upregulated in selected MM cell lines *in vitro* [5,12,15]. Additionally, though not shown in MM, certain members of the MRP1 family (MRP2/canalicular multispecific organic anion transporter [cMOAT], MRP3, and MRP5) have also been shown to mediate clearance of specific chemotherapeutic drugs [16]. The major vault protein lung resistance protein (LRP), a component of nuclear vault ribonucleoproteins (large ribonucleoproteins involved in nuclear–cytoplasmic trafficking), has been demonstrated to mediate resistance to a number of chemotherapeutic agents through a reduction in the nuclear accumulation of drug [12,17,18]. Moreover, LRP was recently identified as a negative prognostic indicator of patient response to low-dose melphalan (L-phenylalanine mustard [L-PAM]) and prednisone treatment in MM [19].

MDR, associated with the aforementioned transporters, has been directly linked with drug efflux both out of the cell and away from drug targets [2,17,20]. However, other molecular determinants have been shown to regulate intracellular drug accumulation at the target [21].

The alkylating agent melphalan is frequently used in MM therapy. Nevertheless, patients become refractory to melphalan and to other alkylating agents. *In vitro* studies have demonstrated that melphalan-selected resistance is associated with a number of determinants involved in drug detoxification (reduced drug accumulation at target cells), including increased glutathione S-transferase (GST) expression, glutathione (GSH) levels, and γ-glutamylcysteine synthase (γ-GCS) activity [4,22,23].

However, more recently, selective resistance to melphalan in MM has been shown to occur independently of GSH-related factors [21]. Harada et al. demonstrated that acquired melphalan resistance was mediated through a reduction in the expression of CD98/4F2hc, a component of the putative L-phenylalanine transporter. Decreased expression of CD98 directly correlated with decreased intracellular melphalan uptake, subsequently reducing drug accumulation at target cells. These findings demonstrate the myriad of MDR determinants that can be acquired by MM cells to reduce chemotherapeutic drug concentration at drug targets.

Alterations in drug targets

Alterations in drug targets are exemplified by changes in the expression and function of DNA topoisomerase II (topo II) and the glucocorticoid receptor (GR) [24–26].

Topo II

Topo II is an ATP-dependent enzyme that moderates the torsional stress placed on the DNA double helix during DNA replication, RNA transcription, chromosomal condensation, and strand separation [27].

Topo IIα and topo IIβ are targets for several classes of chemotherapeutic drugs, termed topo II poisons. Topo II poisons (inhibitors) act through the stabilization of the cleavable complex (DNA-topo II complex), leading to DNA strand breaks and the activation of cell death machinery. Resistance to topo II inhibitors correlates with decreased levels of topo II protein expression via a reduction in transcription, altered protein status, and allelic deletions, as well as decreased enzymatic activity resulting from mutations in specific domains of topo II [22,24,28,29]. Decreased topo II protein expression and loss-of-function mutations reduce topo II inhibitor-mediated DNA damage by reducing the amount of drug target available, thereby lessening DNA strand breaks. Although specific correlations between *in vitro* mechanisms of resistance to topo II inhibitors and clinical resistance in MM have yet to be elucidated [30,31], the historical accuracy of *in vitro* observations suggests that alterations in topo II may remain clinically relevant.

Glucocorticoid receptors

Clinical correlations between *in vitro* selected mechanisms of acquired resistance and glucocorticoids (GCs) have been observed [32,33]. GCs are an integral component of many regimens of MM chemotherapy. However, following an initial response, most patients acquire resistance to hormone therapy.

GC-mediated cytolysis involves the binding of hormones to specific GRs. GRs are latent transcription factors maintained in the cytosol as multimeric protein complexes until they are stimulated by GCs. Upon binding with GCs, GRs enter the nucleus where they bind specific GC response elements and regulate the expression of specific genes that are critical for cellular homeostasis [34–36].

Contrary to the role of GCs in cellular homeostasis, exposure of MM cells to GCs facilitates cell death through the induction and repression of genes implicated in both cell growth and apoptosis [37–40]. Acquired resistance to GC cytotoxicity in MM has been shown to correlate with decreased GR expression, point mutations in the GR gene, and the expression of isoforms lacking the hormone-binding domain (HBD) [26,32,41,42]. Elevated expression of this HBD-deficient GR isoform, termed GR-P, has been observed in MM patients refractory to GC therapy [32]. This indicates that overexpression of GR-P may be a mechanism of acquired MDR in patients with MM.

Antiapoptotic proteins

It is well documented that the cytotoxic effects of therapeutic agents involve activation of the intrinsic apoptotic cascade (see **Figure 1**) [43–47]. Therefore, endogenous inhibitors of apoptotic signaling can affect therapeutic response. Bcl-2 and Bcl-X_L are two antiapoptotic members of the Bcl-2 family of oncogenes capable of attenuating programmed cell death (PCD) mediated by multiple cytotoxic agents in MM [48–51]. Selective expression of one (or both) of these antiapoptotic determinants may be an important mechanism of acquired MDR.

Prevailing dogma suggests that cytotoxic drugs (directly or indirectly) induce disruption of mitochondrial permeability transition, thereby mediating the release of cytochrome c and the activation of downstream caspases. Activated caspases cleave cytosolic, nuclear, and cytoskeletal factors, resulting in the demise of the cell. The antiapoptotic Bcl-2 family members (Bcl-2, Bcl-X_L, Mcl-1) regulate mitochondrial release of cytochrome c and subsequent apoptosis. Therefore, one potential approach to sensitize MM cells to chemotherapy is to modulate expression of either of these antiapoptotic effectors. Bcl-2 antisense, an agent that sensitizes MM cells to cytotoxic stress by downregulating Bcl-2 expression, is currently under investigation in Phase III trials.

A number of reports have demonstrated Bcl-2 expression in MM patient specimens [52,53]. Increased Bcl-2 levels have been shown to correlate with decreased sensitivity to cytotoxic agents – including dexamethasone, doxorubicin, and paclitaxel – in MM cells and patient specimens [49–51]. Exposure of MM cell lines to doxorubicin, etoposide, and hydrogen peroxide selectively stimulated Bcl-2 expression [51], thus further implicating acquired Bcl-2 expression in acquired MDR. Upon secondary (subsequent) exposure, previously treated cells were now resistant to doxorubicin [51].

Although these results highlight the potential role of Bcl-2 in acquired MDR, the significance of Bcl-2 expression in MM patients

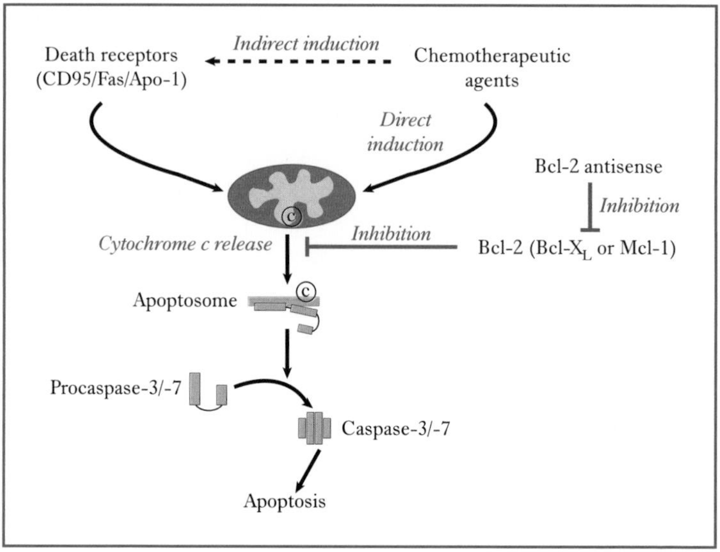

Figure 1. Cytotoxic drugs utilize physiological pathways of cell death and are subject to regulation by endogenous antiapoptotic determinants, such as Bcl-2. Cytotoxic agents induce programmed cell death either directly or via the activation of physiological cell-surface death receptors (eg, CD95/Fas/Apo-1). These death-initiating cascades converge at the mitochondria, mediating the activation of a common death cascade. Targeting the mitochondria stimulates the release of cytochrome c. In turn, cytochrome c facilitates the formation of a protein multimer termed the apoptosome, which is composed of cytochrome c, dATP, apoptosis activating factor-1, and procaspase-9. Apoptosome formation facilitates caspase-9 activation and subsequent cleavage of procaspase-3 and procaspase-7 into effector caspase-3 and caspase-7, respectively. Activated effector caspases target intracellular proteins, promoting the demise of the cell. Bcl-2 and other antiapoptotic family members function by inhibiting the release of cytochrome c from the mitochondria and inhibiting the activation of this common apoptotic cascade. Therefore, therapies such as Bcl-2 antisense oligonucleotides that target Bcl-2 family members may provide a novel means of subverting specific mechanisms of multidrug resistance. Antisense oligonucleotides specific to Bcl-2 bind Bcl-2 mRNA and inhibit the expression of new Bcl-2 protein. In the absence of newly expressed Bcl-2 protein, cellular levels of Bcl-2 are depleted, thereby sensitizing MM cells to chemotherapy.

and in acquired MDR remains incompletely defined. *In vitro*, increased Bcl-X_L expression has been observed in anthracycline-selected MM cell lines. The correlation between Bcl-X_L expression and resistance to anthracyclines suggests that elevated levels of this prosurvival protein may be an important effector of acquired MDR by blocking a key step in the apoptotic cascade common to numerous cytotoxic agents [51]. Furthermore, Bcl-X_L was expressed with a higher incidence in relapsed MM patients than newly diagnosed patients [54], suggesting a correlation between Bcl-X_L levels and the acquisition of MDR *in vivo*.

Together, these studies demonstrate that relative levels of Bcl-2 and Bcl-X_L (and other members of the Bcl-2 family) may be important determinants in acquired MDR, and that the development of novel agents to modulate their expression may effectively sensitize MM cells to conventional therapies.

Other apoptotic-signaling components may also play a role in acquired MDR. Apoptotic signaling from the CD95/Fas/Apo-1 death receptor has been demonstrated to mediate the cytotoxicity of certain drugs [47,55,56], and decreased levels of CD95 have been shown to correlate with increasing doxorubicin-selection pressure of *in vitro* selected MDR MM cell lines [57]. However, the involvement of CD95 in therapy-mediated apoptosis appears to be specific to certain drugs and cell lines [43,45,46,55].

De novo MDR

The BM has long been hypothesized to play a key role in the disease pathology of MM. It is rich in mitogens, growth factors, and adhesive matrices that facilitate MM cell homing and expansion [58–61]. Studies have demonstrated that extrinsic effectors of the BM milieu may directly block cytotoxic stress-mediated MM cell death [6,9,10,62]. The antiapoptotic determinants of the BM consist of both soluble factors and direct MM cell contact (see **Table 2**) [6,9,11,48,62–64]. The identification of these determinants in *de novo* drug insensitivity may provide novel drug targets and,

	Antiapoptotic determinants of the BM				
	Soluble factors			Direct MM cell contact	
	IL-6-mediated pathways	**Insulin-like growth factor-mediated pathways**[1]	**Interferon-α–mediated pathways**	**Integrin-mediated adhesion to fibronectin**	**MM cell adhesion to bone marrow stromal cells**
Mechanisms involved	Ras/Raf–MEK–ERK1/2	Insulin receptor substrate	JAK/STAT3: Bcl-X_L and Mcl-1	Increased levels of $p27^{Kip1}$	Production of IL-6
	Phosphatidylinositol 3-kinase/SHP-2	Ras/MAPK		Intracellular redistribution of topo IIβ	
	JAK/STAT3: Bcl-X_L and Mcl-1			Intracellular redistribution of cFLIPL[1]	
	Jun N-terminal kinase/stress activated kinase[1]				

Table 2. Mechanisms of *de novo* multidrug resistance identified in multiple myeloma (MM). BM: bone marrow; cFLIPL: cellular FLICE-like inhibitory protein-long; ERK: extracellular signal-related kinase; IL: interleukin; JAK: Janus kinase; MAPK: mitogen-activated protein kinase; MEK: MAPK kinase; SHP-2: SH2-containing protein tyrosine phosphatase; STAT3: signal transducer and activator of transcription 3.
[1]Antiapoptotic. However, no direct link to drug resistance has been established.

therefore, lead to the design of new pharmacological agents and regimens for use in MM therapy.

Soluble factors

Historically, MM pathology has been attributed to the host of cytokines and chemokines that are produced at high levels in the microenvironment of the BM [63,65–67]. A number of these soluble factors, including interleukin (IL)-6, insulin-like growth factor (IGF)-1, and interferon (IFN)-α, have been shown to confer resistance to cytotoxic insult [6,63,68–70].

An expanding body of evidence indicates that IL-6 is one of the primary growth and survival factors in MM [6,63,71–73]. Studies have demonstrated that other soluble factors associated with MM, including tumor necrosis factor (TNF)-α, IL-1β, transforming growth factor (TGF)-β, and vascular endothelial growth factor (VEGF), function in part by stimulating the production of IL-6 by BM stromal cells (BMSCs) [34,59,65,74,75].

The prominence of IL-6 in BM in MM has resulted in significant research into characterizing its effects on growth and survival, and elucidating the specific signaling pathways involved [76,77]. The cytokine IL-6 binds to a cell-surface receptor complex consisting of an IL-6-specific transmembrane component (IL-6R) and a larger transmembrane signaling protein common to several cytokine receptor complexes (gp130). IL-6 binding and receptor multimerization facilitates the phosphorylation of gp130 and initiation of three major signaling pathways in MM cells:

- the Ras/Raf–mitogen-activated protein kinase kinase (MEK)–extracellular signal-related kinase (ERK) 1/2 pathway [70–72,78]
- the phosphatidylinositol (PI) 3-kinase pathway [69,79]
- the Janus kinase (JAK)/signal transducer and activator of transcription (STAT) pathway [63]

These pathways have been implicated in IL-6-mediated resistance to both physiological and chemotherapy-mediated apoptosis [6,48,63,73,80,81]. Studies examining the effects of IL-6 in MM survival have been carried out in numerous MM cell lines, resulting in the identification of specific IL-6 signal cascades and antiapoptotic target molecules (see **Figure 2**). The number of antiapoptotic IL-6 targets suggests that a single soluble factor has the potential to regulate drug sensitivity through multiple effectors. In MM cell lines, IGF-1 and IFN-α have been shown to confer resistance to cytotoxic stress independently of IL-6. However, a number of reports have indicated that antiapoptotic signaling from IGF-1 and IFN-α may share downstream effectors with IL-6 [67,68,78].

The Ras/Raf–MEK–ERK1/2 and the JNK/SAPK pathways

The specific antiapoptotic effectors of ERK1/2 phosphorylation have not yet been identified.

The PI 3-kinase pathway

Different effectors of IL-6-mediated drug resistance appear to have different (and in some cases specific) antiapoptotic mechanisms. In MM, resistance to dexamethasone – but not ionizing radiation (IR) or CD95/Fas/Apo-1-induced apoptosis – has been shown to involve phosphorylation (activation) of related focal adhesion tyrosine kinase (RAFTK/Pyk2/CAKβ) [82]. IL-6-mediated resistance to dexamethasone, but not IR or CD95 cross-linking, was subsequently shown to involve phosphatidylinositol (PI) 3-kinase-dependent dephosphorylation of RAFTK via the activation of SH2-containing protein tyrosine phosphatase (SHP-2) [6]. These results indicate that IL-6 signaling via PI 3-kinase and SHP-2 specifically inhibits dexamethasone-mediated PCD through the inactivation of RAFTK/Pyk2/CAKβ.

Although Akt phosphorylation has been linked to MM cell survival, the specific antiapoptotic effectors remain unknown. In other systems, specific antiapoptotic targets of Akt have been identified, including Bad and procaspase-9.

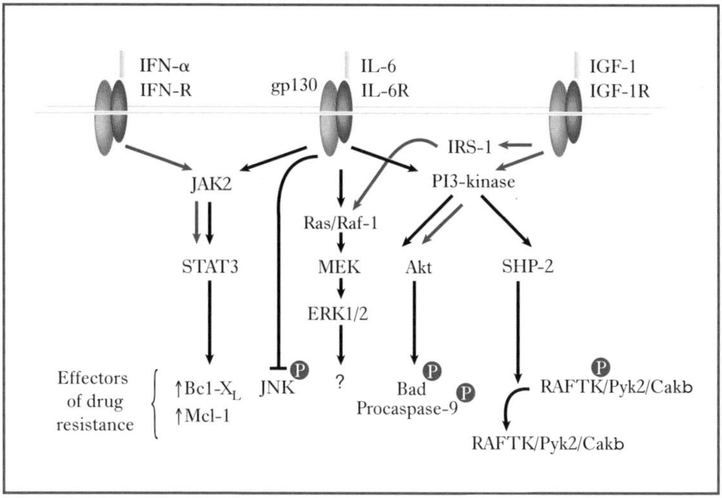

Figure 2. Interferon (IFN)-α, interleukin (IL)-6, and insulin-like growth factor (IGF)-1 signaling cascades confer multidrug resistance in multiple myeloma. ERK1/2: extracellular signal-regulated kinase 1/2; IFN-R: IFN-α receptor; IGF-1R: IGF-1 receptor; IRS-1: insulin receptor substrate-1; JAK2: janus kinase 2; JNK: c-Jun N-terminal kinase; MEK: mitogen-activated protein kinase kinase; Ⓟ : phosphorylated; PI 3-kinase: phosphatidylinositol 3-kinase: RAFTK: related focal adhesion tyrosine kinase; SHP-2: SH2-containing protein tyrosine phosphatase; STAT3: signal transducer and activator of transcription 3.

The JAK/STAT pathway

Activation of JAK/STAT3 signaling following IL-6 ligand–receptor binding has been shown to increase expression of the more global inhibitors of PCD: Bcl-X_L and Mcl-1 [63,67,83,84]. These antiapoptotic proteins have been shown to attenuate PCD mediated by a number of cytotoxic agents in MM [63,67,83].

Direct cell contact

In 1972, Durand and Sutherland were amongst the first to demonstrate that the physical environment in which a cancer cell resides strongly affects cellular sensitivity to cytotoxic stress [85]. Since then, direct contact between cancer cells and their environment has been shown to influence cellular response to both physiological and chemotherapeutic mediators of cell death [10]. Interactions between cells and their physical environment are mediated by a superfamily of glycoprotein transmembrane receptors – cell adhesion molecules (CAMs) – that provide a molecular link between the environment, cellular architecture, and intracellular signaling cascades. These cell-surface receptors include:

- the immunoglobulin family
- cadherins
- selectins
- hyaluronate receptors
- receptor tyrosine phosphatases
- integrins

It has long been proposed that a number of CAMs coordinate homing, lodging, and differentiation of MM cells in the BM through specific homotypic and heterotypic interactions with environmental ligands [86–88]. As with soluble factors associated with MM, interactions between MM cells and extracellular matrix (ECM) components or adjacent cells of the BM confer *de novo* MDR [7–9,11].

Integrin-mediated adhesion

Of the CAM superfamily of proteins, the role of cell survival and MDR has been best characterized in the integrin family of cell-surface receptors. Integrins are a family of single-pass heterodimeric membrane receptors. A number of different α and β subunits have been identified, giving rise to numerous potential heterodimeric receptors with specific ligand-binding properties [89].

Integrin heterodimers specifically bind to extracellular ligands such as fibronectin (FN), vitronectin, laminin, collagens, or other CAMs [89,90]. Affinity for ligand binding is positively or negatively controlled by a host of intracellular signaling factors, or by "inside-out" signaling (from cytoplasm to extracellular domain), often involving small prenylated signaling molecules [91–93]. Integrin receptors lack intrinsic kinase activity and so depend on associated factors such as the scaffold proteins vinculin, talin, and paxillin, and the signaling proteins focal adhesion kinase, RAFTK, PI 3-kinase, and others. This intracellular protein organization facilitates the activation of signaling cascades and cytoskeletal changes following the integrin cross-linking that modulates cell growth, differentiation, migration, and survival [18,90,94].

The survival-promoting effects of integrin-mediated adhesion were first described in studies examining anoikis. Anoikis is a phenomenon that describes the spontaneous apoptosis induced by blocking the adhesion of anchorage-dependent cells to an extracellular matrix [10]. These experiments were some of the first to specifically associate the physical microenvironment and antiapoptosis. The survival-promoting effects of the physical microenvironment have since been demonstrated in hematological cell models [10]. Importantly, cellular adhesion has been demonstrated to confer MDR in MM and other hematological malignancies [9–11,62,95].

Integrin-specific cell adhesion-mediated drug resistance (CAM-DR) in MM was initially described in studies demonstrating that β1-integrin-specific adhesion of the MM cell lines RPMI 8226 and U266 to FN (an abundant BM ECM glycoprotein) conferred resistance to several classes of chemotherapeutic agents [9,11,62,64]. FN adhesion has also been shown to confer melphalan resistance to freshly isolated MM patient cells – as opposed to cells maintained in suspension [96] – suggesting that the MDR phenotype of FN adhesion in MM cell lines is also observed in MM patient cells.

Investigation into the specific determinants of CAM-DR may lead to the development of new therapeutic modalities to circumvent *de novo* MDR. Several studies, described below, have begun to define the cellular determinants of CAM-DR in MM.

Increased $p27^{kip1}$

Adhesion of MM cell lines to the extracellular matrix component FN via the FN integrin receptors VLA-4/α4β1 and VLA-5/α5β1 is currently been utilized to examine the specific role of β1 integrin-containing receptors in CAM-DR in MM. β1 integrin-mediated adhesion to immobilized FN was shown to provide a survival advantage over cell death induced by a panel of cytotoxic agents in hematopoietic cancer cell lines [9,11,62].

Hazlehurst et al. demonstrated that prolonged adhesion (48 hours) of the RPMI 8226 MM cell line to FN resulted in $p27^{kip1}$-dependent resistance to etoposide and cell cycle arrest [11]. This demonstrated a correlation between FN adhesion, regulation of $p27^{kip1}$ protein levels, and MM cell sensitivity to chemotherapeutic drugs.

Intracellular redistribution of topo IIβ

Another mechanism by which CAM-DR has been shown to reduce drug cytotoxicity involves alterations in drug targets. However, unlike the acquired mechanisms affecting the drug target topo II that involve decreased expression or mutations in essential domains, adhesion-mediated alterations involve changes in the subcellular localization of the drug targets [95,97].

Although not reported in MM cells, experiments examining the effects of adhesion on drug cytotoxicity in hematopoietic cancer cells have demonstrated that cellular adhesion protects adhered cells from mitoxantrone- and etoposide-induced DNA double-strand breaks and apoptosis, which are induced by topo II poisons [95]. This integrin-mediated reduction in DNA damage parallels a decrease in topo II enzymatic activity, salt extractability, and altered nuclear localization of topo IIβ. This study suggests that adhesion-mediated alterations in the subcellular localization of key chemotherapeutic targets could be an important regulatory mechanism by which environmental effectors may regulate sensitivity to cytotoxic agents.

Intracellular redistribution of cFLIP$_L$

It has been demonstrated that the intracellular redistribution of the antiapoptotic effector cellular FLICE-like inhibitory protein-long (cFLIP$_L$) – a physiological regulator of CD95-mediated apoptosis – correlates with protection from CD95-mediated apoptosis following adhesion of MM cells to FN [64]. Other cellular models have similarly provided evidence that adhesion-induced trafficking of apoptotic machinery and drug targets correlates with sensitivity to PCD [97,98]. These data, together with evidence of increased p27^{kip1} protein levels, suggest that adhesion-orchestrated changes in the subcellular localization of apoptotic effectors may be an important mechanism by which the physical environment confers resistance to cytotoxic stress and MDR.

The bone marrow microenvironment: a network of survival signals

For the purposes of clarity, we have thus far divided the mechanisms of *de novo* MDR in MM into two categories: soluble mediators of MDR, and MDR mediated by direct contact. However, logic dictates that in the BM these soluble and physical environmental effectors function in concert. With this in mind, a growing number of studies have begun to delineate the complex network of signals that coordinate the protective effects of the BM microenvironment. This network is likely to involve paracrine and autocrine signaling, as well as regulatory events mediated by adhesion of MM cells to BMSCs (see **Figure 3**).

In addition to its antiapoptotic function, adhesion may be an important catalyst in the production of soluble factors. It has been shown that adhesion of MM cells to BMSCs induces BMSC production of IL-6 [99]. IL-6 has also been shown to indirectly increase the adherent potential of MM cell lines to FN via a sequence of events involving the osteoclast-activating chemokine

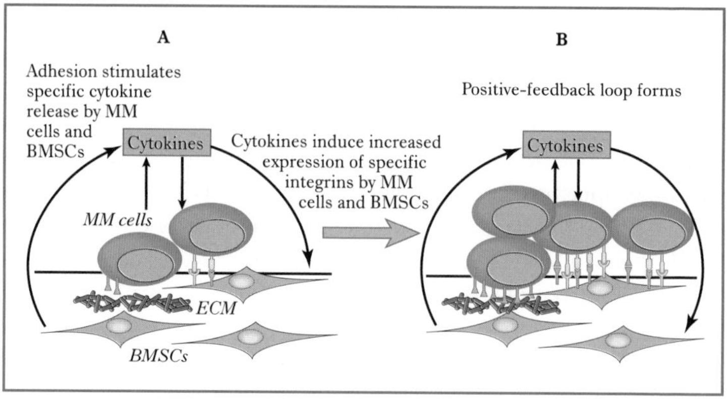

Figure 3. Resident multiple myeloma (MM) cells in the bone marrow may initiate *de novo* multidrug resistance through a network of survival signals. *In vitro* studies have shown that, in the absence of specific environmental effectors, MM cells are sensitive to apoptotic stimuli. In contrast, experiments have demonstrated that MM cells that have been either pretreated with cytokines, or that have adhered to extracellular matrix components or bone marrow stromal cells (BMSCs), are protected from the cytotoxic effects of chemotherapy drugs. **(A)** However, in the context of the bone marrow it is likely that MM cells respond to the adherent and soluble stimuli simultaneously. Moreover, cytokines induce increased expression of specific integrins on MM cells and BMSCs. Adhesion of MM cells also stimulates the expression of specific cytokines by BMSCs and MM cells. **(B)** Therefore, it is likely that both cytokine ligation and the adhesion of MM cells initiate positive-feedback loops that facilitate increased cytokine production and increased adhesion. This network of survival signals may create an environment affording MM cells resistance to chemotherapy. ECM: extracellular matrix.

macrophage inflammatory protein (MIP)-1α [100]. These studies suggest that, in the BM, soluble factors and environmental factors may amplify the effects of one another.

Evidence of this network of soluble and physical BM determinants has been observed in a study demonstrating that coculture of MM cell lines or patient specimens with BMSCs abrogated apoptosis mediated by dexamethasone and all-*trans*-retinoic acid (ATRA) [71].

Honemann et al. showed that treatment with Sant7 – an IL-6 superantagonist – sensitizes cells to dexamethasone and ATRA cytotoxicity, thus demonstrating that the prosurvival effects of BMSCs are at least partly mediated by the production of IL-6. Further evidence for this hypothesis has been shown in studies examining the antiapoptotic nature of specific coculturing conditions between MM cell lines and BMSCs [101]. The degree of mitoxantrone-resistance afforded to MM cells was dependent upon the coculture condition examined. MM cells cocultured with BMSCs – in the absence or presence of intercellular contact with other BMSCs – were protected from mitoxantrone. MM cells cultured alone were unprotected. However, MM cells adhered to BMSCs were significantly more resistant to chemotherapeutic drugs than cells adjacent to BMSCs or maintained in transwells (ie, allowing communication via soluble factors, but not via cell–cell adhesion).

These results suggest the existence of at least two environmental networks elicited by interactions between MM cells and BMSCs:

- a network involving antiapoptotic paracrine and (potentially) autocrine signaling
- a network involving conjunction of soluble and physical effectors, providing a more pronounced survival advantage

A number of potential soluble or adhesive networks have been elucidated. MM-produced VEGF was recently shown to participate in paracrine signaling, with adjacent BMSCs stimulating their own production of IL-6 [102]. In turn, IL-6 has been associated with the increased adherent potential of MM cells [100,102], and adhesion of MM cells to BMSCs has been demonstrated to stimulate IL-6 production by BMSCs [103]. The MM-produced cytokines IL-1β, TGF-β, and TNF-α have also been shown to facilitate BMSC secretion of IL-6 [66,74]. Furthermore, TNF-α has been demonstrated to modulate the expression of specific CAMs on both MM cells and BMSCs, and to increase the number of MM cells able to adhere to BMSCs [65].

Collectively, these results suggest that *de novo* MDR in MM may be mediated through a complex web of communication; soluble factors and direct contact between MM cells and the BM microenvironment function in concert, potentiating the protective effects of the tumor microenvironment. Importantly, these results suggest that the environment of MM cells significantly affects sensitivity to chemotherapy; therapies designed to disrupt specific signaling cascades, ligand–receptor binding, or interactions between cells and the physical environment may be important targets in the circumvention of MDR.

Therapeutic implications

Greater understanding of the mechanisms of drug resistance in MM has led to the development of multiple clinical trials to evaluate the effects of drugs that: (a) interfere with the known mechanisms of drug resistance; and (b) sensitize the cells to cytotoxic chemotherapy. The potential therapeutic modulators of MDR in MM are shown in **Tables 3** and **4**.

Therapies targeting mechanisms of acquired MDR

Reduced drug accumulation at target cells

Most clinical trials aimed at overcoming mechanisms of reduced drug concentration at target cells have involved a combination of cytotoxic chemotherapy with chemosensitizers that act by blocking P-gp function, thus increasing intracellular drug concentrations [104,105]. Several chemosensitizing agents, including verapamil, cyclosporin, dexverapamil, quinine, valspodar (PSC 833), and the acridine derivative GF 12098, have been identified and tested in patients [105–110].

In 1988, clinical use of verapamil was first tested in a patient with advanced MM who was refractory to vincristine, doxorubicin, and pulsed dexamethasone (VAD) chemotherapy; disease stabilization resulted [111]. Since then, the efficacy and toxicity of verapamil, given as a chemosensitizer in combination with VAD chemotherapy, has been examined in both Phase II and Phase III trials. However,

Reduced intracellular drug accumulation at target	Antiapoptotic proteins
Verapamil[1]	Bcl-2 antisense[1]
Cyclosporin A[1]	
Valspodar (PSC-833)[1]	
Quinine[1]	
Dexverapamil	
GF 12098	

Table 3. Potential therapeutic modulators of multidrug resistance (MDR) in multiple myeloma: mechanisms of acquired MDR.
[1]Previously or currently under investigation in clinical trials in MM.

Direct cell contact	Soluble factors
Blocking peptides (RZ-3, HYD-1)	Sant7 (Interleukin-6 receptor super-antagonist)
Prenylation (FTIs, GGTIs)[1]	Ras processing (FTIs, GGTIs)[1]
Isoprenoid biosynthesis (bisphosphonates)[1]	Thalidomide and its derivatives[1]
Thalidomide and its derivatives[1]	Bcl-2 antisense[1]

Table 4. Potential therapeutic modulators of multidrug resistance (MDR) in multiple myeloma: mechanisms of *de novo* MDR. FTIs: farnesyl transferase inhibitors; GGTIs: geranylgeranyl transferase inhibitors.
[1]Previously or currently under investigation in clinical trials in MM.

results have been discouraging due to the cardiac toxicity associated with verapamil at the doses required for P-gp inhibition, and have failed to demonstrate a clinical benefit in the Phase III trial [106].

Cyclosporin has also been tested as a P-gp modulator in MM. Whilst it was able to reverse MDR in some patients, responses were of a short duration, and the neurotoxicity and myelosuppression associated with vincristine and doxorubicin, respectively, were enhanced [107,108]. Valspodar (PSC 833) –

a cyclosporin D analog – has been developed in an attempt to produce novel chemosensitizers with increased safety and efficacy [110,112]. In a Phase I study, a total of 22 MM patients who were refractory to VAD or melphalan were treated with three cycles of VAD plus an escalating dose of valspodar [113]. The dose-limiting toxicities were myelosuppression and neuropathy, and dose reduction was necessary in almost half of the patients. A partial response was seen in 45% of patients.

Several Phase III trials are currently investigating the efficacy of valspodar in patients with MM, acute myelogenous leukemia, myelodysplasia, and non-Hodgkin's lymphoma. These trials should determine the role of P-gp in conferring clinical drug resistance in patients with MM and other hematological malignancies.

Antiapoptotic proteins

In an attempt to target the mechanisms of drug resistance associated with inhibition of drug-induced apoptosis, a multicenter randomized clinical trial is currently being conducted. Relapsed patients with MM are randomized to receive high-dose dexamethasone, either alone or in combination with Bcl-2 antisense. The aim of this trial is to determine the relevance of Bcl-2 expression as a mediator of dexamethasone resistance in MM. It should also provide a clinical account for the use of antisense therapy in targeting other genes involved in MM drug resistance.

As described previously and depicted in **Figure 2**, genes involved in IL-6 signal transduction, such as Ras/Erk signaling and/or JAK/STAT3 signaling, are other potential targets. Targeting these pathways may inhibit disease progression and sensitize the cells to conventional chemotherapy.

Therapies targeting mechanisms of *de novo* MDR

De novo MDR can be conferred through interactions between MM cells and the BM microenvironment. Adhesion of MM cells to BMSCs triggers the secretion of cytokines, which augment the growth, survival, and resistance to chemotherapy of MM cells [102]. Specifically, adhesive interaction of MM cells with BMSCs renders MM cells resistant to multiple cytotoxic drugs.

It is hypothesized that drugs capable of disrupting the interactions between MM cells and BMSCs could result in improved chemotherapy response rates and longer overall survival times. Drugs that have been shown to act by altering MM intercellular interactions include thalidomide, thalidomide derivatives, and bisphosphonates [114–122].

Thalidomide and derivatives

Thalidomide and its derivatives have been shown to alter the profile of BM adhesion molecules and to immunomodulate the BM microenvironmental cytokine milieu by changing the profile of the adhesion molecule or cytokine secretions such as IL-6, TNF-α, and VEGF, thereby rendering the MM cells more sensitive to dexamethasone [114]. Clinically, thalidomide in combination with dexamethasone has been shown to be more effective than either agent alone [115,116].

Bisphosphonates

Similarly, bisphosphonates have been proposed to inhibit the release of MM growth factors by BMSCs [117,118]. The aminobisphosphonates have been shown to inhibit adhesion of breast and prostate cancer cells to FN [119]. However, it has been shown *in vivo* (murine model) that MM cell treatment with aminobisphosphonates interferes with the homing of MM cells to the BM [117]. Furthermore, preliminary *in vitro* data have revealed that bisphosphonates reverse MM cell adhesion to FN. These studies indicate that bisphosphonates inhibit MM cell adhesion and, therefore, may be good candidate drugs to circumvent *de novo* MDR.

From a clinical perspective, bisphosphonates have shown efficacy in preventing skeletal-related events and prolonging survival in MM patients who fail to respond to first-line therapy [54]. A randomized clinical trial is currently being

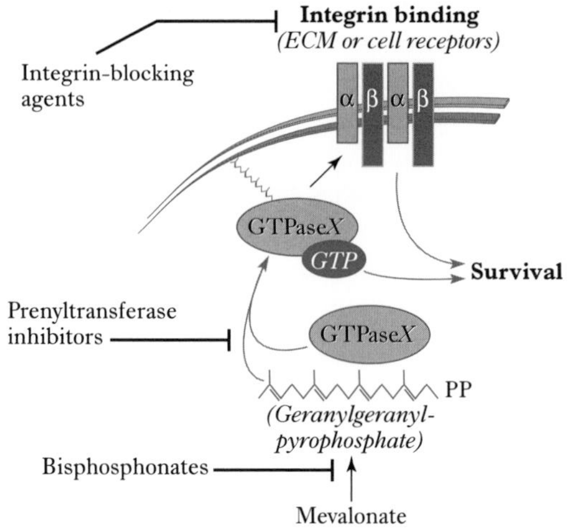

Figure 4. Novel candidates for circumventing cell adhesion-mediated drug resistance. ECM: extracellular matrix.

conducted to examine the effects of bisphosphonates, given concomitantly with chemotherapy, on *de novo* MDR. The objective of this trial is to determine whether treatment with the aminobisphosphonate zoledronate immediately prior to chemotherapy enhances response to treatment – ie, increases complete response rates.

Other agents

Other agents that may interfere with myeloma–stromal cell interactions, such as prenyltransferase inhibitors or integrin-blocking agents (peptides) (see **Figure 4**), are currently undergoing preclinical testing in both *in vitro* and *in vivo* systems [54,117,123–126]. These studies may lead to clinical trials that will examine the effect of these agents on *de novo* MDR.

Several biochemical processes involved in the regulation of cellular adhesion, and potentially CAM-DR, are subject to modulation by novel pharmacological agents. A number of reports have demonstrated that prenylated small GTPases regulate integrin–ligand affinity. To this end, compounds that block prenyl modification of these proteins (eg, farnesyl transferase inhibitors and geranylgeranyl transferase inhibitors) or isoprenoid synthesis (eg, bisphosphonates) are potential therapeutics that may disrupt cell–environment interactions.

Furthermore, inhibition of prenylation may also affect other prosurvival cascades involving Ras, such as those mediated by interleukin (IL)-6 or other soluble factors. Abrogation of cellular contact and/or IL-6 signaling may in turn sensitize cancer cells to cytotoxic insult, thereby preventing *de novo* MDR and subsequent emergence of acquired MDR, facilitating more successful cancer treatment.

Conclusion

Acquired and *de novo* MDR have been presented as two individual phenomena. However, this does not exclude the idea that these two determinants of MDR may be more intimately linked.

In 1990, it was shown that drug selection *in vivo* differed from selection *in vitro* [7]. In support of these findings, studies demonstrated that drug selection in MM cell lines correlated with an increased adherent potential through increased integrin expression and "inside out" signaling of integrin receptors [9,62]. Together, these reports suggest that during the MDR selection process, cells may utilize (or require) mechanisms of *de novo* MDR to overcome initial drug cytotoxicity, and that this transient antiapoptotic state may allow for the acquisition of genetic mechanisms of MDR. In turn, the development of drugs that target *de novo* MDR may concomitantly compromise the acquisition of MDR.

Further understanding of the molecular events involved in the development of drug resistance in MM may lead to significant therapeutic interventions with drugs (individually or in combination) that target the different mechanisms involved.

References

1. Kyle RA. Multiple myeloma. Diagnostic challenges and standard therapy. *Semin Hematol* 2001;38(2 Suppl. 3):11S–24S.
2. Dalton WS, Durie BG, Alberts DS et al. Characterization of a new drug-resistant human myeloma cell line that expresses P-glycoprotein. *Cancer Res* 1986;46:5125–30.
3. Bhalla K, Huang Y, Tang C et al. Characterization of a human myeloid leukemia cell line highly resistant to taxol. *Leukemia* 1994;8:465–75.
4. Bellamy WT, Dalton WS, Gleason MC et al. Development and characterization of a melphalan-resistant human multiple myeloma cell line. *Cancer Res* 1991;51:995–1002.
5. Ross DD. Novel mechanisms of drug resistance in leukemia. *Leukemia* 2000;14:467–73.
6. Chauhan D, Pandey P, Hideshima T et al. SHP2 mediates the protective effect of interleukin-6 against dexamethasone-induced apoptosis in multiple myeloma cells. *J Biol Chem* 2000;275:27845–50.
7. Teicher BA, Herman TS, Holden SA et al. Tumor resistance to alkylating agents conferred by mechanisms operative only *in vivo*. *Science* 1990;247:1457–61.
8. Sethi T, Rintoul RC, Moore SM et al. Extracellular matrix proteins protect small cell lung cancer cells against apoptosis: a mechanism for small cell lung cancer growth and drug resistance *in vivo*. *Nat Med* 1999;5:662–8.
9. Damiano JS, Cress AE, Hazlehurst LA et al. Cell adhesion mediated drug resistance (CAM-DR): role of integrins and resistance to apoptosis in human myeloma cell lines. *Blood* 1999;93:1658–67.
10. Shain KH, Dalton WS. Cell adhesion is a key determinant in *de novo* multidrug resistance (MDR): new targets for the prevention of acquired MDR. *Mol Cancer Ther* 2001;1:69–78.
11. Hazlehurst LA, Damiano JS, Buyuksal I et al. Adhesion to fibronectin via beta 1 integrins regulates p27kip1 levels and contributes to cell adhesion mediated drug resistance (CAM-DR). *Oncogene* 2000;19:4319–27.
12. Wyler B, Shao Y, Schneider E et al. Intermittent exposure to doxorubicin *in vitro* selects for multifactorial non-P-glycoprotein-associated multidrug resistance in RPMI 8226 human myeloma cells. *Br J Haematol* 1997;97:65–75.
13. Hazlehurst LA, Foley NE, Gleason-Guzman MC et al. Multiple mechanisms confer drug resistance to mitoxantrone in the human 8226 myeloma cell line. *Cancer Res* 1999;59:1021–8.
14. Kartner N, Riordan JR, Ling V. Cell surface P-glycoprotein associated with multidrug resistance in mammalian cell lines. *Science* 1983;221:1285–8.
15. Futscher BW, Foley NE, Gleason-Guzman MC et al. Verapamil suppresses the emergence of P-glycoprotein-mediated multi-drug resistance. *Int J Cancer* 1996;66:520–5.
16. Scheffer GL, Kool M, Heijn M et al. Specific detection of multidrug resistance proteins MRP1, MRP2, MRP3, MRP5, and MDR3 P-glycoprotein with a panel of monoclonal antibodies. *Cancer Res* 2000;60:5269–77.
17. Scheffer GL, Schroeijers AB, Izquierdo MA et al. Lung resistance-related protein/major vault protein and vaults in multidrug-resistant cancer. *Curr Opin Oncol* 2000;12:550–6.
18. Rimsza LM, Campbell K, Dalton WS et al. The major vault protein (MVP), a new multidrug resistance associated protein, is frequently expressed in multiple myeloma. *Leuk Lymphoma* 1999;34:315–24.
19. Raaijmakers HG, Izquierdo MA, Lokhorst HM et al. Lung-resistance-related protein expression is a negative predictive factor for response to conventional low but not to intensified dose alkylating chemotherapy in multiple myeloma. *Blood* 1998;91:1029–36.

20. Abbaszadegan MR, Cress AE, Futscher BW et al. Evidence for cytoplasmic P-glycoprotein location associated with increased multidrug resistance and resistance to chemosensitizers. *Cancer Res* 1996;56:5435–42.
21. Harada N, Nagasaki A, Hata H et al. Down-regulation of CD98 in melphalan-resistant myeloma cells with reduced drug uptake. *Acta Haematol* 2000;103:144–151.
22. Glisson BS, Sullivan DM, Gupta R et al. Mediation of multi-drug resistance in a Chinese hamster ovary cell line by a mutant type II topoisomerase. *NCI Monogr* 1987:89–93.
23. Mulcahy RT, Bailey HH, Gipp JJ. Up-regulation of gamma-glutamylcysteine synthetase activity in melphalan-resistant human multiple myeloma cells expressing increased glutathione levels. *Cancer Chemother Pharmacol* 1994;34:67–71.
24. Valkov NI, Sullivan DM. Drug resistance to DNA topoisomerase I and II inhibitors in human leukemia, lymphoma, and multiple myeloma. *Semin Hematol* 1997;34(4 Suppl. 5):48S–62S.
25. Friche E, Danks MK, Schmidt CA et al. Decreased DNA topoisomerase II in daunorubicin-resistant Ehrlich ascites tumor cells. *Cancer Res* 1991;51:4213–8.
26. Moalli PA, Pillay S, Weiner D et al. A mechanism of resistance to glucocorticoids in multiple myeloma: transient expression of a truncated glucocorticoid receptor mRNA. *Blood* 1992;79:213–22.
27. Austin CA, Marsh KL. Eukaryotic DNA topoisomerase II beta. *Bioessays* 1998;20:215–26.
28. Wang H, Jiang Z, Wong YW et al. Decreased CP-1 (NF-Y) activity results in transcriptional down-regulation of topoisomerase IIalpha in a doxorubicin-resistant variant of human multiple myeloma RPMI 8226. *Biochem Biophys Res Commun* 1997;237:217–24.
29. Feldhoff PW, Mirski SE, Cole SP et al. Altered subcellular distribution of topoisomerase II alpha in a drug-resistant human small cell lung cancer cell line. *Cancer Res* 1994;54:756–62.
30. Wilson CS, Medeiros LJ, Lai R et al. DNA topoisomerase II alpha in multiple myeloma: a marker of cell proliferation and not drug resistance. *Mod Pathol* 2001;14:886–91.
31. Ishikawa H, Kawano MM, Okada K et al. Expressions of DNA topoisomerase I and II gene and the genes possibly related to drug resistance in human myeloma cells. *Br J Haematol* 1993;83:68–74.
32. Krett NL, Pillay S, Moalli PA et al. A variant glucocorticoid receptor messenger RNA is expressed in multiple myeloma patients. *Cancer Res* 1995;55:2727–9.
33. Moalli PA, Pillay S, Krett NL et al. Alternatively spliced glucocorticoid receptor messenger RNAs in glucocorticoid-resistant human multiple myeloma cells. *Cancer Res* 1993;53:3877–9.
34. Cole TJ, Blendy JA, Monaghan AP et al. Targeted disruption of the glucocorticoid receptor gene blocks adrenergic chromaffin cell development and severely retards lung maturation. *Genes Dev* 1995;9:1608–21.
35. Planey SL, Litwack G. Glucocorticoid-induced apoptosis in lymphocytes. *Biochem Biophys Res Commun* 2000;279:307–12.
36. Smith MR, Xie T, Joshi I et al. Dexamethasone plus retinoids decrease IL-6/IL-6 receptor and induce apoptosis in myeloma cells. *Br J Haematol* 1998;102:1090–7.
37. Chauhan D, Auclair D, Robinson EK et al. Identification of genes regulated by dexamethasone in multiple myeloma cells using oligonucleotide arrays. *Oncogene* 2002;21:1346–58.
38. Robertson NM, Bodine PV, Hsu TC et al. Modulator inhibits nuclear translocation of the glucocorticoid receptor and inhibits glucocorticoid-induced apoptosis in the human leukemic cell line CEM C-7. *Cancer Res* 1995;55:548–56.

39. Hardin J, MacLeod S, Grigorieva I et al. Interleukin-6 prevents dexamethasone-induced myeloma cell death. *Blood* 1994;84:3063–70.
40. Kool M, van der LM, de Haas M et al. MRP3, an organic anion transporter able to transport anti-cancer drugs. *Proc Natl Acad Sci USA* 1999;96:6914–9.
41. Karkera JD, Taymans SE, Turner G et al. Deletion of a consensus oestrogen response element half-site in the glucocorticoid receptor of human multiple myeloma. *Br J Haematol* 1997;99:372–4.
42. de Lange P, Segeren CM, Koper JW et al. Expression in hematological malignancies of a glucocorticoid receptor splice variant that augments glucocorticoid receptor-mediated effects in transfected cells. *Cancer Res* 2001;61:3937–41.
43. Landowski TH, Shain KH, Oshiro MM et al. Myeloma cells selected for resistance to CD95-mediated apoptosis are not cross-resistant to cytotoxic drugs: evidence for independent mechanisms of caspase activation. *Blood* 1999;94:265–74.
44. Shain KH, Landowski TH, Buyuksal I et al. Clonal variability in CD95 expression is the major determinant in Fas-medicated, but not chemotherapy-medicated apoptosis in the RPMI 8226 multiple myeloma cell line. *Leukemia* 2000;14:830–40.
45. Eischen CM, Kottke TJ, Martins LM et al. Comparison of apoptosis in wild-type and Fas-resistant cells: chemotherapy-induced apoptosis is not dependent on Fas/Fas ligand interactions. *Blood* 1997;90:935–43.
46. Kaufmann SH, Earnshaw WC. Induction of apoptosis by cancer chemotherapy. *Exp Cell Res* 2000;256:42–9.
47. Friesen C, Herr I, Krammer PH et al. Involvement of the CD95 (APO-1/FAS) receptor/ligand system in drug-induced apoptosis in leukemia cells. *Nat Med* 1996;2:574–7.
48. Oshiro MM, Landowski TH, Catlett-Falcone R et al. Inhibition of JAK kinase activity enhances Fas-mediated apoptosis but reduces cytotoxic activity of topoisomerase II inhibitors in U266 myeloma cells. *Clin Cancer Res* 2001;7:4262–71.
49. Gazitt Y, Rothenberg ML, Hilsenbeck SG et al. Bcl-2 overexpression is associated with resistance to paclitaxel, but not gemcitabine, in multiple myeloma cells. *Int J Oncol* 1998;13:839–48.
50. Gazitt Y, Fey V, Thomas C et al. Bcl-2 overexpression is associated with resistance to dexamethasone, but not melphalan, in multiple myeloma cells. *Int J Oncol* 1998;13:397–405.
51. Tu Y, Xu FH, Liu J et al. Upregulated expression of BCL-2 in multiple myeloma cells induced by exposure to doxorubicin, etoposide, and hydrogen peroxide. *Blood* 1996;88:1805–12.
52. Harada N, Hata H, Yoshida M et al. Expression of Bcl-2 family of proteins in fresh myeloma cells. *Leukemia* 1998;12:1817–20.
53. Brown RD, Pope B, Luo XF et al. The oncoprotein phenotype of plasma cells from patients with multiple myeloma. *Leuk Lymphoma* 1994;16:147–56.
54. Tu Y, Renner S, Xu F et al. BCL-X expression in multiple myeloma: possible indicator of chemoresistance. *Cancer Res* 1998;58:256–62.
55. Fulda S, Sieverts H, Friesen C et al. The CD95 (APO-1/Fas) system mediates drug-induced apoptosis in neuroblastoma cells. *Cancer Res* 1997;57:3823–9.
56. Aragane Y, Kulms D, Metze D et al. Ultraviolet light induces apoptosis via direct activation of CD95 (Fas/APO-1) independently of its ligand CD95L. *J Cell Biol* 1998;140:171–82.
57. Landowski TH, Gleason-Guzman MC, Dalton WS. Selection for drug resistance results in resistance to Fas-mediated apoptosis. *Blood* 1997;89:1854–61.
58. Ferlin M, Noraz N, Hertogh C et al. Insulin-like growth factor induces the survival and proliferation of myeloma cells through an interleukin-6-independent transduction pathway. *Br J Haematol* 2000;111:626–34.

59. Dankbar B, Padro T, Leo R et al. Vascular endothelial growth factor and interleukin-6 in paracrine tumor-stromal cell interactions in multiple myeloma. *Blood* 2000;95:2630–6.
60. Podar K, Tai YT, Davies FE et al. Vascular endothelial growth factor triggers signaling cascades mediating multiple myeloma cell growth and migration. *Blood* 2001;98:428–35.
61. Urashima M, Ogata A, Chauhan D et al. Interleukin-6 promotes multiple myeloma cell growth via phosphorylation of retinoblastoma protein. *Blood* 1996;88:2219–27.
62. Damiano JS, Dalton WS. Integrin-mediated drug resistance in multiple myeloma. *Leuk Lymphoma* 2000;38:71–81.
63. Catlett-Falcone R, Landowski TH, Oshiro MM et al. Constitutive activation of STAT3 signaling confers resistance to apoptosis in human U266 myeloma cells. *Immunity* 1999;10:105–15.
64. Shain KH, Landowski TH, Dalton WS. Adhesion-mediated intracellular redistribution of c-Fas-associated death domain-like IL-1-converting enzyme-like inhibitory protein-long confers resistance to CD95-induced apoptosis in hematopoietic cancer cell lines. *J Immunol* 2002;168:2544–53.
65. Hideshima T, Chauhan D, Schlossman R et al. The role of tumor necrosis factor alpha in the pathophysiology of human multiple myeloma: therapeutic applications. *Oncogene* 2001;20:4519–27.
66. Choi SJ, Cruz JC, Craig F et al. Macrophage inflammatory protein 1-alpha is a potential osteoclast stimulatory factor in multiple myeloma. *Blood* 2000;96:671–5.
67. Jourdan M, De Vos J, Mechti N et al. Regulation of Bcl-2-family proteins in myeloma cells by three myeloma survival factors: interleukin-6, interferon-alpha and insulin-like growth factor 1. *Cell Death Differ* 2000;7:1244–52.
68. Ferlin-Bezombes M, Jourdan M, Liautard J et al. IFN-alpha is a survival factor for human myeloma cells and reduces dexamethasone-induced apoptosis. *J Immunol* 1998;161:2692–9.
69. Tu Y, Gardner A, Lichtenstein A. The phosphatidylinositol 3-kinase/AKT kinase pathway in multiple myeloma plasma cells: roles in cytokine-dependent survival and proliferative responses. *Cancer Res* 2000;60:6763–70.
70. Xu FH, Sharma S, Gardner A et al. Interleukin-6-induced inhibition of multiple myeloma cell apoptosis: support for the hypothesis that protection is mediated via inhibition of the JNK/SAPK pathway. *Blood* 1998;92:241–51.
71. Honemann D, Chatterjee M, Savino R et al. The IL-6 receptor antagonist SANT-7 overcomes bone marrow stromal cell-mediated drug resistance of multiple myeloma cells. *Int J Cancer* 2001;93:674–80.
72. Ogata A, Chauhan D, Teoh G et al. IL-6 triggers cell growth via the Ras-dependent mitogen-activated protein kinase cascade. *J Immunol* 1997;159:2212–21.
73. Lichtenstein A, Tu Y, Fady C et al. Interleukin-6 inhibits apoptosis of malignant plasma cells. *Cell Immunol* 1995;162:248–55.
74. Urashima M, Ogata A, Chauhan D et al. Transforming growth factor-beta1: differential effects on multiple myeloma versus normal B cells. *Blood* 1996;87:1928–38.
75. Chauhan D, Uchiyama H, Akbarali Y et al. Multiple myeloma cell adhesion-induced interleukin-6 expression in bone marrow stromal cells involves activation of NF-kappa B. *Blood* 1996;87:1104–12.
76. Iwasaki T, Hamano T, Ogata A et al. Clinical significance of interleukin-6 gene expression in the bone marrow of patients with multiple myeloma. *Int J Hematol* 1999;70:163–8.
77. Grigorieva I, Thomas X, Epstein J. The bone marrow stromal environment is a major factor in myeloma cell resistance to dexamethasone. *Exp Hematol* 1998;26:597–603.

78. Ogawa M, Nishiura T, Oritani K et al. Cytokines prevent dexamethasone-induced apoptosis via the activation of mitogen-activated protein kinase and phosphatidylinositol 3-kinase pathways in a new multiple myeloma cell line. *Cancer Res* 2000;60:4262–9.
79. Hideshima T, Nakamura N, Chauhan D et al. Biologic sequelae of interleukin-6 induced PI3-K/Akt signaling in multiple myeloma. *Oncogene* 2001;20:5991–6000.
80. Chauhan D, Kharbanda S, Ogata A et al. Interleukin-6 inhibits Fas-induced apoptosis and stress-activated protein kinase activation in multiple myeloma cells. *Blood* 1997;89:227–34.
81. Frassanito MA, Cusmai A, Iodice G et al. Autocrine interleukin-6 production and highly malignant multiple myeloma: relation with resistance to drug-induced apoptosis. *Blood* 2001;97:483–9.
82. Chauhan D, Hideshima T, Pandey P et al. RAFTK/PYK2-dependent and -independent apoptosis in multiple myeloma cells. *Oncogene* 1999;18:6733–40.
83. Puthier D, Bataille R, Amiot M. IL-6 up-regulates mcl-1 in human myeloma cells through JAK / STAT rather than ras/MAP kinase pathway. *Eur J Immunol* 1999;29:3945–50.
84. Puthier D, Derenne S, Barille S et al. Mcl-1 and Bcl-xL are co-regulated by IL-6 in human myeloma cells. *Br J Haematol* 1999;107:392–5.
85. Sutherland RM, Durand RE. Cell contact as a possible contribution to radiation resistance of some tumours. *Br J Radiol* 1972;45:788–9.
86. Uchiyama H, Barut BA, Chauhan D et al. Characterization of adhesion molecules on human myeloma cell lines. *Blood* 1992;80:2306–14.
87. Pellat-Deceunynck C, Barille S, Puthier D et al. Adhesion molecules on human myeloma cells: significant changes in expression related to malignancy, tumor spreading, and immortalization. *Cancer Res* 1995;55:3647–53.
88. Barker HF, Ball J, Drew M et al. The role of adhesion molecules in multiple myeloma. *Leuk Lymphoma* 1992;8:189–96.
89. Kumar CC. Signaling by integrin receptors. *Oncogene* 1998;17:1365–73.
90. Miyamoto S, Katz BZ, Lafrenie RM et al. Fibronectin and integrins in cell adhesion, signaling, and morphogenesis. *Ann N Y Acad Sci* 1998;857:119–29.
91. Kinashi T, Katagiri K, Watanabe S et al. Distinct mechanisms of alpha 5beta 1 integrin activation by Ha-Ras and R-Ras. *J Biol Chem* 2000;275:22590–6.
92. Keely PJ, Rusyn EV, Cox AD et al. R-Ras signals through specific integrin alpha cytoplasmic domains to promote migration and invasion of breast epithelial cells. *J Cell Biol* 1999;145:1077–88.
93. Katagiri K, Hattori M, Minato N et al. Rap1 is a potent activation signal for leukocyte function-associated antigen 1 distinct from protein kinase C and phosphatidylinositol-3-OH kinase. *Mol Cell Biol* 2000;20:1956–69.
94. Clark EA, Brugge JS. Integrins and signal transduction pathways: the road taken. *Science* 1995;268:233–9.
95. Hazlehurst LA, Valkov N, Wisner L et al. Reduction in drug-induced DNA double-strand breaks associated with beta1 integrin-mediated adhesion correlates with drug resistance in U937 cells. *Blood* 2001;98:1897–903.
96. Painter JS, Hazlehurst LA, Shain KS et al. *De novo* drug resistance associated with cell adhesion protects myeloma cells from melphalan induced cytotoxicity: comparison of de novo and acquired mechanisms of resistance in myeloma cells. *Blood* 2001;98:2987A (Abstr.).
97. Oloumi A, MacPhail SH, Johnston PJ et al. Changes in subcellular distribution of topoisomerase II alpha correlate with etoposide resistance in multicell spheroids and xenograft tumors. *Cancer Res* 2000;60:5747–53.
98. Gilmore AP, Metcalfe AD, Romer LH et al. Integrin-mediated survival signals regulate the apoptotic function of Bax through its conformation and subcellular localization. *J Cell Biol* 2000;149:431–46.

99. Uchiyama H, Barut BA, Mohrbacher AF et al. Adhesion of human myeloma-derived cell lines to bone marrow stromal cells stimulates interleukin-6 secretion. *Blood* 1993;82:3712–20.
100. Alsina M, Gerbino E, Painter JS et al. The effects of interleukin-6 on myeloma cell adhesion to fibronectin are mediated by macrophage inflammatory protein 1-alpha. *Blood* 2001;98:2666A (Abstr.).
101. Nefedova Y, Landowski TH, Dalton WS. Bone marrow stromal-derived soluble factors and direct cell contact contribute to *de novo* drug resistance of myeloma cells by distinct mechanisms. *Leukemia* 2003;17:1175–82.
102. Gupta D, Treon SP, Shima Y et al. Adherence of multiple myeloma cells to bone marrow stromal cells upregulates vascular endothelial growth factor secretion: therapeutic applications. *Leukemia* 2001;15:1950–61.
103. Chauhan D, Uchiyama H, Urashima M et al. Regulation of interleukin 6 in multiple myeloma and bone marrow stromal cells. *Stem Cells* 1995;13(Suppl. 2):35–9.
104. Sonneveld P. Multidrug resistance in haematological malignancies. *J Intern Med* 2000;247:521–34.
105. Dalton WS, Jove R. Drug resistance in multiple myeloma: approaches to circumvention. *Semin Oncol* 1999;26(5 Suppl. 13):23S–27S.
106. Dalton WS, Crowley JJ, Salmon SS et al. A phase III randomized study of oral verapamil as a chemosensitizer to reverse drug resistance in patients with refractory myeloma. A Southwest Oncology Group study. *Cancer* 1995;75:815–20.
107. Pilarski LM, Yatscoff RW, Murphy GF et al. Drug resistance in multiple myeloma: cyclosporin A analogues and their metabolites as potential chemosensitizers. *Leukemia* 1998;12:505–9.
108. Sonneveld P, Suciu S, Weujermans P et al. Cyclosporin A combined with vincristine, doxorubicin and dexamethasone (VAD) compared with VAD alone in patients with advanced refractory multiple myeloma: an EORTC-HOVON randomized phase III study (06914). *Br J Haematol* 2001;115:895–902.
109. Lehnert M, Dalton WS, Roe D et al. Synergistic inhibition by verapamil and quinine of P-glycoprotein-mediated multidrug resistance in a human myeloma cell line model. *Blood* 1991;77:348–54.
110. Jonsson B, Nilsson K, Nygren P et al. SDZ PSC-833 – a novel potent *in vitro* chemosensitizer in multiple myeloma. *Anticancer Drugs* 1992;3:641–6.
111. Durie BG, Dalton WS. Reversal of drug-resistance in multiple myeloma with verapamil. *Br J Haematol* 1988;68:203–6.
112. Tai HL. Technology evaluation: Valspodar, Novartis AG. *Curr Opin Mol Ther* 2000;2:459–67.
113. Sonneveld P, Marie JP, Huisman C et al. Reversal of multidrug resistance by SDZ PSC 833, combined with VAD (vincristine, doxorubicin, dexamethasone) in refractory multiple myeloma. A phase I study. *Leukemia* 1996;10:1741–50.
114. Singhal S, Mehta J, Desikan R et al. Antitumor activity of thalidomide in refractory multiple myeloma. *N Engl J Med* 1999;341:1565–71.
115. Palumbo A, Giaccone L, Bertola A et al. Low-dose thalidomide plus dexamethasone is an effective salvage therapy for advanced myeloma. *Haematologica* 2001;86:399–403.
116. Dimopoulos MA, Zervas K, Kouvatseas G et al. Thalidomide and dexamethasone combination for refractory multiple myeloma. *Ann Oncol* 2001;12:991–5.
117. Cruz JC, Alsina M, Craig F et al. Ibandronate decreases bone disease development and osteoclast stimulatory activity in an *in vivo* model of human myeloma. *Exp Hematol* 2001;29:441–7.
118. Boissier S, Ferreras M, Peyruchaud O et al. Bisphosphonates inhibit breast and prostate carcinoma cell invasion, an early event in the formation of bone metastases. *Cancer Res* 2000;60:2949–54.

119. Boissier S, Magnetto S, Frappart L et al. Bisphosphonates inhibit prostate and breast carcinoma cell adhesion to unmineralized and mineralized bone extracellular matrices. *Cancer Res* 1997;57:3890–4.
120. Hideshima T, Chauhan D, Shima Y et al. Thalidomide and its analogs overcome drug resistance of human multiple myeloma cells to conventional therapy. *Blood* 2000;96:2943–50.
121. Davies FE, Raje N, Hideshima T et al. Thalidomide and immunomodulatory derivatives augment natural killer cell cytotoxicity in multiple myeloma. *Blood* 2001;98:210–6.
122. Rajkumar SV. Current status of thalidomide in the treatment of cancer. *Oncology (Huntingt)* 2001;15:867–74. Discussion: 877–9.
123. Wang E, Casciano CN, Clement RP et al. The farnesyl protein transferase inhibitor SCH66336 is a potent inhibitor of MDR1 product P-glycoprotein. *Cancer Res* 2001;61:7525–9.
124. Andela VB, Rosenblatt JD, Schwarz EM et al. Synergism of aminobisphosphonates and farnesyl transferase inhibitors on tumor metastasis. *Clin Orthop* 2002;397:228–39.
125. Johnston SR, Kelland LR. Farnesyl transferase inhibitors – a novel therapy for breast cancer. *Endocr Relat Cancer* 2001;8:227–35.
126. DeRoock IB, Pennington ME, Sroka TC et al. Synthetic peptides inhibit adhesion of human tumor cells to extracellular matrix proteins. *Cancer Res* 2001;61:3308–13.

3

Novel biological therapies

Paul G Richardson, Teru Hideshima,
& Kenneth C Anderson

Introduction

Despite conventional-dose and high-dose therapies, multiple myeloma (MM) remains incurable, and novel biological treatment approaches are required. Many studies have characterized the molecular mechanisms by which MM cell–host bone marrow (BM) interactions regulate tumor cell growth, survival, and migration in the BM milieu.

Current lines of investigation have led to the discovery of novel therapies to improve patient outcome based upon targeting both the MM cell and the BM microenvironment [1]. To achieve this goal, systems have been developed for studying growth, survival, and drug resistance mechanisms intrinsic to MM cells, both *in vitro* and in animal models *in vivo*. Investigators have sought to characterize mechanisms of MM cell homing to the BM, as well as factors that promote MM cell growth, survival, drug resistance, and migration in the BM microenvironment (eg, MM cell–BM stromal cell [BMSC] interactions, cytokines, and angiogenesis) [2].

These model systems have permitted the study of several promising therapies that can target the MM cell in the BM microenvironment and thereby overcome classical drug resistance *in vitro*. Therapeutic agents include thalidomide and its more potent immunomodulatory drug (IMiD) analogs [3], the novel first-in-class proteasome inhibitor bortezomib (formerly known as PS-341) [4], and arsenic trioxide (As_2O_3) (see **Figure 1**) [5]. Other promising agents include vascular endothelial growth

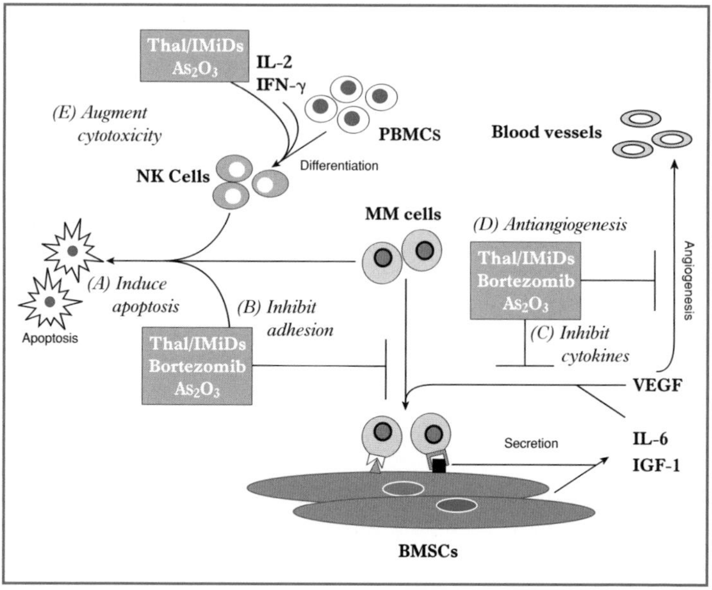

Figure 1. Novel biological therapies targeting multiple myeloma (MM) cells and the bone marrow (BM) microenvironment. Specifically, these agents: **(A)** induce apoptosis or G1 growth arrest in drug-resistant MM cell lines and patient cells; **(B)** modulate MM cell binding to BM stromal cells (BMSCs); **(C)** block induction of cytokine secretion (eg, insulin-like growth factor [IGF]-1, interleukin [IL]-6, vascular endothelial growth factor [VEGF]) triggered by MM cell binding to BMSCs; **(D)** inhibit angiogenesis; and **(E)** augment natural killer (NK) cell activity against autologous MM cells, thus inducing anti-MM immunity. As_2O_3: arsenic trioxide; IMiDs: immunomodulatory drugs; Thal: thalidomide.

factor (VEGF) inhibitors, TRAIL/Apo2L humanized monoclonal antibody, and 2-methoxyestradiol (2ME2) [2].

Once the *in vitro* success of these novel agents has been demonstrated, their efficacy is then tested in murine models. For example, thalidomide (3-amino-phthalimido-glutarimide), the IMiDs, and bortezomib inhibit human MM cell growth, decrease associated angiogenesis, and prolong host survival in a model where human MM cells and a matrix gel are injected subcutaneously into severe combined immunodeficiency (SCID) mice [2]. These laboratory studies have been translated into Phase I and II trials to evaluate their clinical utility and toxicity. IMiDs and bortezomib have already demonstrated marked clinical anti-MM activity, even in patients with refractory, relapsed MM, confirming the utility of the preclinical models in helping to identify and validate novel therapeutic agents [3,6,7]. Moreover, the success of bortezomib in heavily pretreated patients with advanced MM has led to its recent approval by the US Food and Drug Administration (FDA) for the treatment of patients whose disease has progressed despite two prior lines of therapy. This represents a landmark in drug development, going from bench studies to bedside approval in only 3 years [7].

In vitro gene array studies with conventional and novel therapies (eg, dexamethasone and bortezomib, respectively) have helped to establish genomic patterns associated with both treatment response and drug resistance [2]. Thus, samples obtained from patients treated with these drugs may help to identify *in vivo* targets and mechanisms of novel drug action against drug resistance mechanisms, and might also aid in determining whether the *in vivo* targets of these novel therapies correlate with those implicated in their *in vitro* anti-MM activity.

On aggregate, these *in vitro* and *in vivo* studies have demonstrated the critical role of evaluating the MM cell in its BM microenvironment to elucidate MM pathogenesis, understand resistance, and identify novel therapeutic targets.

Potential targets

The signaling cascades involved in the cytokine-mediated proliferation, survival, drug resistance, and migration of MM cells have been characterized (see **Figure 2**). For example, certain cytokines (eg, interleukin [IL]-6 and VEGF) trigger proliferation of MM cells via mitogen-activated protein kinase (MAPK) signaling, whereas MM cell migration induced by cytokines (eg, VEGF) is mediated via a protein kinase C (PKC)-dependent,

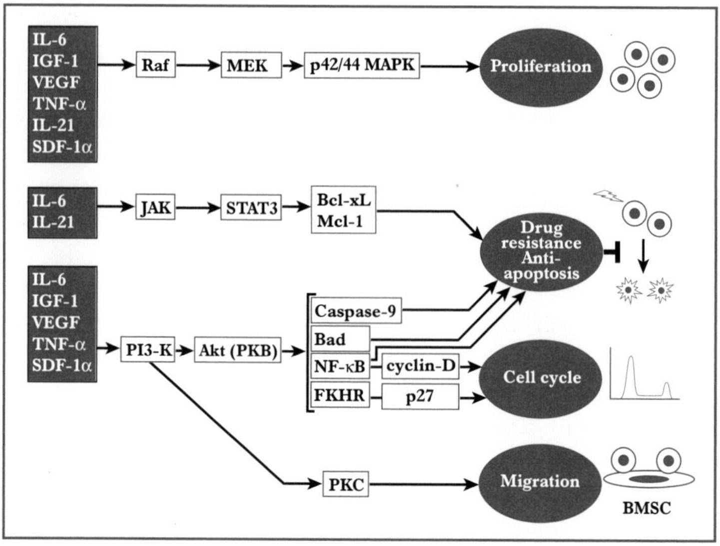

Figure 2. Apoptotic signaling cascades mediating growth, survival, and migration in multiple myeloma (MM) cells. Proliferation of MM is mediated via the Raf/MEK/p42/44 mitogen activated protein kinase (MAPK) pathway. Survival (drug resistance) is mediated via the Janus kinase (JAK)/signal transducer and activator of transcription (STAT)3 pathway, and upregulation of Bcl-xL and Mcl-1. Antiapoptosis is also mediated by phosphatidylinositol (PI)3-kinase (K)/Akt (protein kinase [PK] B]) signaling, with downstream activation of Bad and nuclear factor (NF)-κB, and/or inactivation of caspase-9. NF-κB and FKHR (forkhead in rhabdomyosarcoma) modulate cyclin D and p27^{Kip1}, thereby regulating cell cycle progression. Signaling via PI3-K induces downstream PKC activity and MM cell migration. BMSC: bone marrow stromal cell; IGF: insulin-like growth factor; IL: interleukin; TNF: tumor necrosis factor; SDF-1α: stromal-cell-derived factor-1α; VEGF: vascular endothelial growth factor. Reprinted by permission from *Nature Reviews Cancer* 2002;2:927–37 copyright 2004 Macmillan Magazines Ltd.

extracellular signal-related kinase (ERK)-independent pathway [2]. Fas-, γ-irradiation (IR)-, and dexamethasone-induced MM cell apoptosis is mediated by distinct signaling cascades [2]. Dexamethasone-triggered (but not IR- or Fas-triggered) apoptosis is mediated via activation of related adhesion focal tyrosine kinase (RAFTK) [2]. Dexamethasone-mediated MM apoptosis is not associated with mitochondrial cytochrome c release, but is mediated by second mitochondrial activator of caspase (Smac) release [2]. Furthermore, cytosolic Smac disrupts the X-linked inhibitor of apoptosis protein (XIAP)/caspase-9 complex, thereby allowing activation of caspase-9, cleavage of caspase-3, and apoptosis to follow. Whilst dexamethasone activates caspase-9, novel agents such as thalidomide and other IMiDs deactivate caspase-8 and downstream cascades, including caspase-3 [2]. This construct supports the utility of successfully coupling novel and conventional treatments, such as thalidomide and dexamethasone [8].

Mechanisms of drug resistance induced by cytokines have been identified: IL-6 and insulin-like growth factor (IGF)-1 inhibit apoptosis triggered by dexamethasone (but not IR) via Akt signaling and nuclear factor (NF)-κB activation, with downstream induction of intracellular inhibitors of apoptosis (IAPs), including FLICE (Fas-associated death domain-like interleukin-1β-converting enzyme) inhibitor protein (FLIP), survivin, cellular inhibitor-of-apoptosis protein (cIAP)-2, *A1/bfl-1*, and XIAP, as well as specific activation of SH2-containing protein tyrosine phosphatase SHP-2, thereby blocking activation of RAFTK [2,9]. These studies validate signaling cascades triggered by MM localization in the BM microenvironment mediating tumor cell growth, survival, drug resistance, and migration as possible sites of therapeutic opportunity using small molecule inhibitors.

Therapeutic agents

Thalidomide and IMiDs (also see Chapter 4)

Thalidomide is a derivative of glutamic acid, and inhibits tumor necrosis factor (TNF)-α production [10–12] and angiogenesis by blocking basic fibroblast growth factor and/or VEGF [13–15]. Reports of increased BM angiogenesis in MM [16,17], coupled with the antiangiogenic properties of thalidomide [10], provided the empiric rationale for its use in the treatment of MM, and clinical responses were observed in nearly one-third of patients with relapsed MM refractory to conventional chemotherapy [18,19].

Therapy	Effect on signaling cascades			
	MEK/MAPK	JAK/STAT3	PI 3-kinase/Akt	NF-κB
Thalidomide/ IMiDs	+	–	–	+
Bortezomib	+	–	–	+
As_2O_3	–	+	–	+

Table 1. Effect of novel therapies on IL-6-induced signaling cascades in multiple myeloma cells. As_2O_3: arsenic trioxide; IMiDs: immunomodulatory drugs; JAK: Janus kinase; MAPK: mitogen activated protein kinase; MEK: MAPK kinase; NF: nuclear factor; PI: phosphatidylinositol; STAT: signal transducer and activator of transcription; –: no effect; +: inhibitory effect. Reprinted by permission from *Nature Reviews Cancer* 2002;2:927–37 copyright 2004 Macmillan Magazines Ltd.

However, preclinical studies demonstrate that thalidomide and the more potent IMiDs have additional mechanisms of anti-MM activity. These include direct pro-apoptotic effects on MM cells, inhibition of adhesion of MM cells to BMSCs, decreased secretion of key growth factors (such as IL-6) from the BM milieu, and immune-modulation resulting in increased natural killer (NK) cell activity (see **Figure 1**) [20].

The precise molecular mechanisms by which thalidomide and the IMiDs mediate these elements of anti-MM activity remain to be fully defined. However, some important mechanisms have been elucidated. The effect on IL-6-induced signaling cascades in MM cells is shown in **Table 1**. This results in:

- inhibition of growth and MAPK activity induced by cytokines such as IL-6 and IGF-1
- inhibition of NF-κB activation and its sequelae (including up-regulation of adhesion molecules on MM cells and BMSCs, and increased binding with related increased cytokine secretion)
- blockade of VEGF-induced PKC-dependent MM cell migration

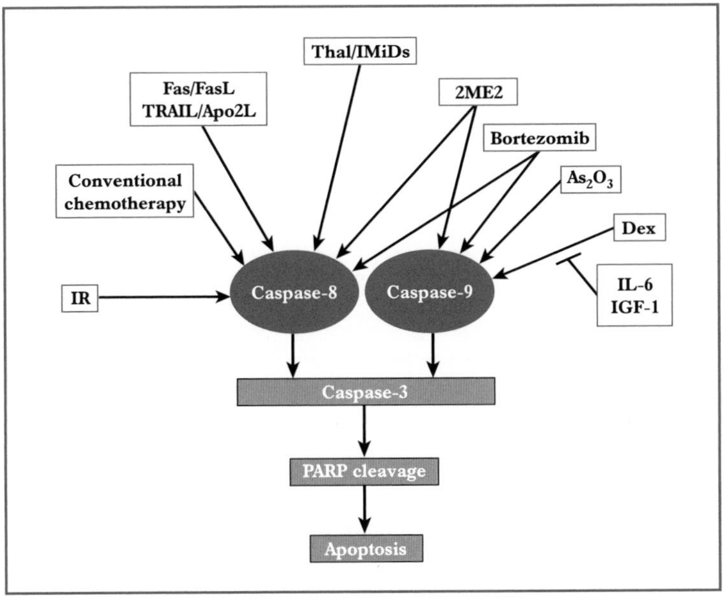

Figure 3. Apoptotic signaling pathways triggered by conventional chemotherapy and novel therapies. Fas/FasL, γ-radiation (IR), tumor necrosis factor-related apoptosis-inducing ligand (TRAIL), and thalidomide (Thal)/immunomodulatory drugs (IMiDs) trigger caspase-8, whereas arsenic trioxide (As_2O_3) and dexamethasone (Dex) trigger caspase-9 activation. Bortezomib induces both caspase-8 and caspase-9 activation. Interleukin (IL)-6 and insulin-like growth factor (IGF)-1 activate the phosphatidylinositol (PI)3-kinase/Akt cascade, which inhibits caspase-9/caspase-3 apoptotic signaling. Poly(ADP-ribose) polymerase (PARP) cleavage by caspase-3 leads to apoptosis. 2ME2: 2-methoxyestradiol. Reprinted by permission from *Nature Reviews Cancer* 2002;2:927–37 copyright 2004 Macmillan Magazines Ltd.

IMiDs predominantly trigger caspase-8 apoptotic signaling, and enhance both caspase-8-mediated MM cell apoptosis triggered by Fas or TNF-related apoptosis-inducing ligand (TRAIL) (see **Figure 3**), as well as caspase-9-mediated MM cell killing triggered by dexamethasone [21–23]. Thalidomide and the IMiDs also augment *in vitro* and *in vivo* NK activity against patient MM cells, induce apoptosis, inhibit tumor-associated angiogenesis, and prolong host survival in SCID mice bearing human MM cells [24,25].

Based upon these promising preclinical studies, a Phase I study of Celgene Corp.'s Revlimid (also known as lenalidomide or CC-5013) has been completed in 25 patients with relapsed, refractory MM [3]. Reversible myelosuppression was seen, but the significant constipation, somnolence, and neuropathy typically associated with the use of thalidomide were not observed in this clinical study. Anti-MM clinical activity – evidenced by a >25% decrease in MM serum paraprotein levels – was achieved in two-thirds of the 24 evaluable patients, with stabilization or a decrease in paraprotein level evident in 79% of patients. Based on this promising anti-MM activity and a favorable side-effect profile, Phase II trials are ongoing and Phase III trials have begun in order to better define the clinical utility of lenalidomide in patients with relapsed MM. Studies of lenalidomide as a maintenance therapy are also in development.

Proteasome inhibition

Bortezomib (formerly PS-341)

The ubiquitin–proteasome pathway is a proteolytic system in both the cytosol and nucleus that regulates cyclin and cyclin-dependent kinase inhibitor proteins, thereby regulating cell cycle progression [26]. Bortezomib (pyrazylcarbonyl-Phe-Leu-boronate) represents a first-in-class of peptide boronate proteasome inhibitors of 26S proteasome activity [27]. Bortezomib has been shown to:

- induce, in murine models, marked *in vivo* antitumor activity against human prostate cancer, Burkitt's lymphoma, and adult T cell leukemia [28–30]
- produce additive growth delays against Lewis lung carcinoma when coupled with 5-fluorouracil, cisplatin, taxol, and doxorubicin [31]
- demonstrate antiangiogenic activity in an orthotopic pancreatic cancer model [32]

Proteasome inhibition – and specifically bortezomib – represents a second class of therapeutics targeting the MM cell in its BM

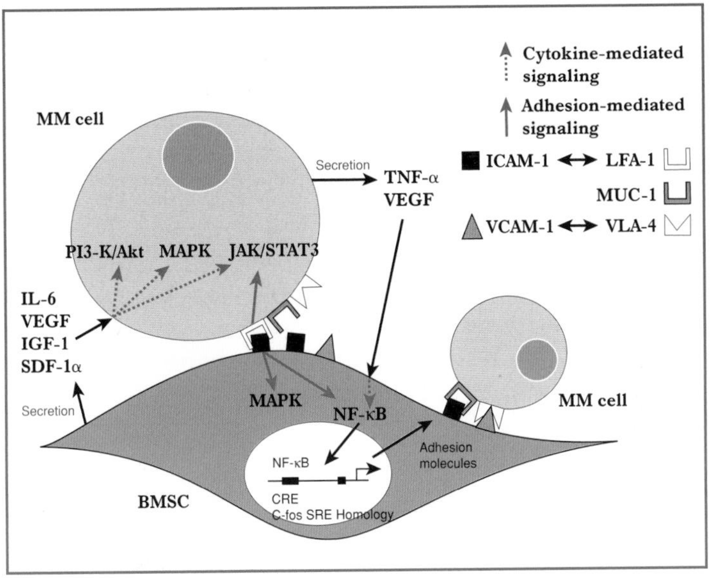

Figure 4. Interaction of multiple myeloma (MM) cells and their bone marrow (BM) milieu. Binding of MM cells to BM stromal cells (BMSCs) via ICAM-1, VCAM-1, and their receptors triggers adhesion- and cytokine-mediated MM cell growth, survival, drug resistance, and migration. MM cell binding to BMSCs induces activation of p42/44 mitogen activated protein kinase (MAPK) and nuclear factor (NF)-κB in BMSCs. Activation of NF-κB upregulates adhesion molecules on both MM cells and BMSCs. Cytokines (tumor necrosis factor [TNF]-α, vascular endothelial growth factor [VEGF]) secreted from MM cells induce interleukin (IL)-6 secretion and NF-κB activation. Cytokines (IL-6, VEGF, insulin-like growth factor [IGF]-1, stromal-cell-derived factor [SDF]-1α) secreted from BMSCs activate major signaling pathways (p42/44 MAPK, Janus kinase [JAK]/STAT3, and/or phosphatidylinositol [PI]3-kinase [K]/Akt) and their downstream targets. CRE: cyclin AMP response element; SRE: serum response element. Reprinted by permission from *Nature Reviews Cancer* 2002;2:927–37 copyright 2004 Macmillan Magazines Ltd.

microenvironment. Based upon studies in which IL-6 has been shown to be the major growth and survival factor for human MM cells, and the observation that MM cell adhesion to BMSCs triggers the transcription and secretion of IL-6 in BMSCs via an

NF-κB-dependent mechanism, it is hypothesized that the blockade of NF-κB using bortezomib may mediate anti-MM activity by inhibiting paracrine IL-6 production in BMSCs (see **Figure 4**) [13,33].

Studies confirm that bortezomib acts directly on MM cells to induce apoptosis of MM cells resistant to known conventional therapies, overcomes the protective effects of IL-6, and adds to the anti-MM effects of dexamethasone (see **Figure 1**) [7]. In the BM microenvironment, bortezomib actively inhibits the binding of MM cells to BMSCs, the transcription and secretion of IL-6 triggered by the adhesion of MM cells to BMSCs, and BM angiogenesis.

Gene microarray profiling studies demonstrate that bortezomib induces transcriptional down-regulation of growth and survival signaling pathways, as well as up-regulation of apoptotic cascades, ubiquitin/proteasome pathways, and expression of heat-shock proteins [34]. One study suggests that bortezomib inhibits DNA repair by cleavage of DNA-dependent protein kinase catalytic subunit [35]. This bioactivity may have important clinical applications, since treatment of MM cell lines resistant to DNA-damaging agents (eg, melphalan, anthracycline) with those agents to which they are resistant, followed 12–24 hours later with sublethal doses of bortezomib, can inhibit DNA repair, overcome drug resistance, and restore sensitivity to DNA-damaging agents [36].

These studies, coupled with a Phase I study of bortezomib in hematologic cancers that demonstrated promising clinical activity in a subset of patients treated with relapsed MM, provided the rationale for a multicenter Phase II trial of bortezomib in MM [37].

Bortezomib treatment in 202 heavily pretreated [7] patients with refractory, relapsed MM demonstrated complete response (CR) and near CR utilizing the rigorous EBMT/Bladé criteria [38] in 10%, with 4% immunofixation-negative and 6% with residual MM paraprotein detectable only by immunofixation. The overall response rate (minimal response + partial response [PR] + CR) was 35%, with an additional 24% experiencing stable disease. Median time to progression [TTP] on bortezomib alone was 7 months and the median duration of survival was 16 months, with a median duration of response of 12 months in those patients with PR and CR. Importantly, the median TTP in all 202 patients on their penultimate regimen prior to entering the trial was 3 months, making the improved TTP seen especially noteworthy [7]. A landmark survival analysis showed that survival for patients with CR and PR after two cycles of bortezomib was significantly better than for nonresponders ($P = 0.007$) [7].

Responses were associated with improved hemoglobin levels, decreased blood transfusion requirements, improvement in renal function, and normalization of uninvolved immunoglobulins. Drug-related gastrointestinal toxicity, transient thrombocytopenia and neutropenia, peripheral neuropathy, and fatigue were the most common side effects seen. Drug-related toxicities were manageable in most cases and neuropathy occurred primarily in patients in whom these conditions were pre-existent, with serious adverse events relatively uncommon [7]. A smaller, randomized Phase II trial ($N = 52$) comparing 1.0 mg/m^2 twice a week for 2 weeks followed by 1 week of rest with the standard 1.3 mg/m^2 according to the same schedule confirmed the activity of bortezomib in both dose arms, but suggested a possible dose–response effect with a higher response rate for the 1.3 mg/m^2 arm, and less toxicity with the lower dose [39].

Based upon this promising clinical activity and tolerable toxicity profile in patients with advanced disease, bortezomib has been approved by the FDA for heavily pretreated patients with MM. It is now undergoing evaluation in Phase II trials to treat patients at earlier stages (eg, newly diagnosed patients), and has been compared with dexamethasone in a multicenter, international Phase III trial of patients with relapsed MM, with completion in October 2003.

Arsenic trioxide

Arsenic trioxide (As_2O_3) modulates cell growth and differentiation of acute promyelocytic leukemia (APL) cells *in vitro*, and induces complete remission in patients with relapsed and refractory APL [40]. Although its growth inhibitory effect in APL is mediated by promyelocytic leukemia (PML) and/or PML-retinoic acid receptor-α fusion protein, As_2O_3 also induces tumor cell apoptosis and down-regulates *Bcl-2* [41,42].

Studies show that As_2O_3 has the following effects [43]:

- it induces apoptosis in drug-resistant MM cell lines and patient cells via caspase-9 activation (see **Figure 3**)
- it inhibits activation of Janus kinase (JAK)/signal transducers and activators of transcription (STAT)3 (see **Table 1**), and induces up-regulation of *Mcl*-1 triggered by IL-6
- it inhibits NF-κB activation in the BM microenvironment, thereby down-regulating adhesion molecule expression and tumor cell–BMSC binding, as well as inhibiting paracrine IL-6 and VEGF transcription and secretion in BMSCs (see **Figures 1** and **4**)

Deaglio et al. reported that As_2O_3 increases the killing of MM cells mediated by lymphokine-activated killer (LAK) cells via selective up-regulation of CD38 and CD54 on MM cells, as well as CD31 and CD11a on LAK cells [44]. Preliminary analysis of data from Phase I and II trials of As_2O_3 in patients with refractory or relapsed MM shows minor decreases or stabilization in MM paraprotein levels. Side effects include leukopenia, anemia, abdominal pain, diarrhea, fever, and fatigue [5]. Another report demonstrates that As_2O_3-induced MM cell cytotoxicity is enhanced by ascorbic acid [45]. Based upon *in vitro* studies showing that dexamethasone enhances As_2O_3-induced MM cell apoptosis [43], a Phase II clinical trial of this combination therapy is ongoing.

VEGF inhibitors

Due to the increased angiogenesis seen in MM, the BM role of VEGF in MM has been characterized [46–48]. VEGF is expressed and secreted by MM cells and BMSCs, and augments IL-6 secretion in BMSCs (see **Figure 4**) [48–50]. MM cells and plasma cell leukemia cells express the high-affinity VEGF receptor Flt-1. VEGF triggers the phosphorylation of Flt-1 and downstream p42/44 MAPK activation and cell proliferation (see **Figure 2**), which is inhibited by anti-VEGF antibody or the MEK inhibitor PD98059 [46].

VEGF induces migration of MM cells, which is abrogated by the PKC inhibitor bisindolylmaleimide I hydrochloride. In addition, VEGF triggers activation of phosphatidylinositol (PI) 3-kinase/Akt. Coupled with β1-integrin-mediated binding to fibronectin, PI 3-kinase triggers recruitment and activation of PKC-α, thereby further enhancing the migration of MM cells [46]. Conversely, the VEGF receptor tyrosine kinase inhibitor PTK787/ZK222584 blocks VEGF-induced tyrosine phosphorylation of Flt-1, MEK/MAPK activation and proliferation, as well as PKC activation-dependent migration [51]. These studies both define VEGF as a novel therapeutic target and provide the basis for a clinical trial – due to begin soon – of PTK787/ZK222584 in patients with relapsed MM.

TRAIL/Apo2L

TRAIL/Apo2 ligand (Apo2L) is a member of the TNF superfamily of death-inducing ligands, which includes TNF-α and Fas ligand (FasL). It binds to cell surface receptors death receptor 4 and death receptor 5, thereby inducing downstream caspase-8-mediated apoptosis of human MM cell lines and patient MM cells that are resistant to conventional therapies (see **Figure 3**) [21,52]. TRAIL/Apo2L also inhibits growth of S6B45 human MM cells in SCID mice [21]. These preclinical studies have provided the rationale for inducing TRAIL apoptotic signaling to overcome drug resistance in MM, and a Phase I study is underway.

2-Methoxyestradiol

A natural metabolite of estradiol, 2ME2 demonstrates potent antitumor and antiangiogenic activity in leukemic cells *in vitro* and *in vivo* [53,54]. It binds poorly to the estrogen receptor, and mediates its antiproliferative effects independently of estrogen receptor expression or responsiveness. It has been demonstrated that 2ME2 inhibits growth and induces apoptosis in drug-resistant MM cell lines and patient cells, enhances dexamethasone-induced apoptosis, overcomes the protective effect of IL-6 and IGF-1, and decreases secretion of VEGF and IL-6 in BMSCs triggered by MM cell binding [55,56]. MM cell apoptosis is induced by 2ME2 via the release of mitochondrial cytochrome c and Smac, followed by activation of caspases-8, -9, and -3 (see **Figure 3**). Based upon these preclinical studies, 2ME2 is under evaluation in MM in a Phase II clinical trial.

Farnesyltransferase inhibitors

The cytosolic enzyme farnesyltransferase transfers the farnesyl group from farnesyl diphosphate to the CAAX motif (C = cysteine, A_1 and A_2 = aliphatic amino acids, X = any amino acid) of *ras*, thereby facilitating its attachment to the inner plasma cell membrane and related signal transduction [57]. Inhibition of farnesylation is a strategy for blocking *ras* activity, and several farnesyltransferase inhibitors inhibit tumor cell growth both *in vitro* and *in vivo* [58]. Cytokine (IL-6, VEGF, IGF-1)-induced proliferation of MM cells is mediated via *ras*/Raf/MAPK signaling [9,46,59], providing the basis for ongoing Phase I and II clinical trials of two promising farnesyltransferase inhibitors: SCH-66336 and R115777 [60,61].

Histone deacetylase inhibitors

Histone acetylation modulates gene expression, cellular differentiation, and cell survival. It is regulated by the opposing activities of histone acetyltransferases and histone deacetylases. Novel hydroxamic acid-based hybrid polar compounds (eg, suberoylanilide hydroxamic acid [SAHA]) are histone deacetylase inhibitors. They induce accumulation of acetylated core nucleosomal histones, with related induction of differentiation and/or apoptosis in transformed and neoplastic cells. It has been shown that SAHA induces growth arrest and apoptosis in MM patient cells and cell lines, irrespective of resistance to dexamethasone or conventional chemotherapy [62]. Since Phase I studies have documented that SAHA is well tolerated, it is a promising novel agent for the treatment of refractory MM. A Phase II study of SAHA in MM is now in progress.

Heat shock protein 90 inhibitors

Heat shock protein (Hsp)90 is a molecular chaperone interacting with target intracellular proteins to facilitate intracellular trafficking, conformational maturation, and 3D folding, all of which are required for correct functioning of the protein. The ansamycin-based antibiotic geldanamycin (GA) and its analogs bind to the critical ATP-binding site of Hsp90, thereby abrogating its chaperoning activity in the MM BM milieu by decreasing IGF-1 receptor and IL-6 receptor expression by MM cells, depleting growth kinases (eg, Akt, inhibitory-κB kinase, and raf) and antiapoptotic proteins (eg, FLIP, XIAP, cIAP, and telomerase), and inhibiting both constitutive and cytokine-induced activation of NF-κB and telomerase in the BM milieu [34]. GA and other Hsp90 inhibitors induce apoptosis of MM cell lines and patient cells that are resistant to dexamethasone, anthracyclines, thalidomide, IMiDs, TRAIL/Apo2L, and bortezomib. Gene microarray profiling shows that bortezomib induces Hsp90 expression in MM cells (see **Table 2**). Conversely, blocking this response with GA enhances MM cell apoptosis triggered by bortezomib. These data, coupled with the observed *in vivo* anti-MM activity of GA in a SCID mouse model, provide the framework for a clinical trial in MM, and one is currently in development.

Future directions

In vitro and animal model studies have demonstrated the importance of the BM in promoting MM cell growth, survival,

	Transcriptional changes						
Caspase cascade	↑ Procaspase-9, -7, and -5	↑ Fas (Apo1, CD95)	↑ DR5 Apo2L/ TRAIL receptor	↑ Fas (trans-membrane)	↓ Soluble (decoy) Fas (alternative splicing)	↓ Toso (negative Fas regulator)	↓ Caspase inhibitors
IGF signaling	↓ IGF-1	↓ IGF-1 receptor	↓ Insulin receptor substrate-1				
I-κB	↑ I-κB kinase-α	↑ I-κB kinase-γ					
Ubiquitin/ proteasome pathway	↑ Ubiquitin	↑ p40.5, p44.5, p55, p58	↑ HsN3, HsC7-I, HsC10-II	↑ p112, p97	↑ Nin1p		
Molecular chaperones	↑ hsp90	↑ hsp70	↑ hsp40	↑ hsp28	↑ hsp32 (heme oxygenase-1)	↑ hsp apg-1	↑ Mitochondrial hsp75

Table 2. Gene microarray profile of transcriptional changes in bortezomib-treated multiple myeloma cells [34]. DR: death receptor; hsp: heat shock protein; HsC: human proteasome subunit C; HsN: human proteasome subunit N; IGF: insulin-like growth factor; I-κB: inhibitory-κB; TRAIL: tumor necrosis factor-related apoptosis-inducing ligand. ↑: up-regulation of transcription; ↓: down-regulation of transcription.

drug resistance, and migration in the BM microenvironment. Promising therapies have been derived, based upon targeting the MM cell in its BM milieu. These studies provide the framework for the development of a new treatment paradigm in MM that targets both the tumor cell and its microenvironment in order to counter this disease, which, despite advances in cytotoxic therapy and transplant, remains incurable.

Novel biological treatment strategies targeting both the tumor cell and its microenvironment can overcome resistance to current therapies, and represent a promising treatment paradigm for improving patient outcome. Many of these agents have multiple biologic activities, which may be advantageous since common fundamental molecular targets – as have been therapeutically exploited in chronic myelocytic leukemia [63] or APL [64] – are lacking in MM.

Ongoing gene microarray and proteomic studies of these novel agents in MM are delineating molecular mechanisms of drug sensitivity versus drug resistance. These studies will derive more selective therapies for validation in animal models and, hopefully, subsequent translation to the bedside through clinical trials. Conversely, gene microarray and proteomic studies of tumor, blood, and BM samples from patients treated in clinical trials of novel agents will define *in vivo* targets conferring drug sensitivity and resistance, and will also provide the framework for the development of more selective, potent, and less toxic next-generation targeted therapies. These studies will also establish the preclinical rationale for combining novel and conventional therapies, and will allow for the selection of those patients most likely to respond.

References

1. Anderson KC. Targeted therapy for multiple myeloma. *Semin Hematol* 2001; 38:286–94.
2. Hideshima T, Anderson KC. Molecular mechanisms of novel therapeutic approaches for multiple myeloma. Nat Rev Cancer *2002;2:927–37.*

3. Richardson P, Schlossman RL, Weller E et al. Immunomodulatory drug CC-5013 overcomes drug resistance and is well tolerated in patients with relapsed multiple myeloma. *Blood* 2002;100:3063–7.
4. Hideshima T, Richardson P, Chauhan D et al. The proteasome inhibitor PS-341 inhibits growth, induces apoptosis, and overcomes drug resistance in human multiple myeloma cells. *Cancer Res* 2001;61:3071–6.
5. Hussein MA. Arsenic trioxide: a new immunomodulatory agent in the management of multiple myeloma. *Med Oncol* 2001;18:239–42.
6. Rajkumar SV, Gertz MA, Kyle RA et al. Current therapy for multiple myeloma. *Mayo Clin Proc* 2002;77:813–22.
7. Richardson PG, Barlogie B, Berenson J et al. A Phase 2 study of bortezomib in relapsed, refractory myeloma. *N Engl J Med* 2003;348:2609–17.
8. Chauhan D, Kharbanda S, Ogata A et al. Interleukin-6 inhibits Fas-induced apoptosis and stress-activated protein kinase activation in multiple myeloma cells. *Blood* 1997;89:227–34.
9. Ogata A, Chauhan D, Teoh G et al. IL-6 triggers cell growth via the Ras-dependent mitogen-activated protein kinase cascade. *J Immunol* 1997;159:2212–21.
10. Sampaio EP, Sarno EN, Galilly R et al. Thalidomide selectively inhibits tumor necrosis factor alpha production by stimulated human monocytes. *J Exp Med* 1991;173:699–703.
11. Moreira AL, Sampaio EP, Zmuidzinas A et al. Thalidomide exerts its inhibitory action on tumor necrosis factor alpha by enhancing mRNA degradation. *J Exp Med* 1993;177:1675–80.
12. Sampaio EP, Kaplan G, Miranda A et al. The influence of thalidomide on the clinical and immunologic manifestation of erythema nodosum leprosum. *J Infect Dis* 1993;168:408–14.
13. D'Amato RJ, Loughnan MS, Flynn E et al. Thalidomide is an inhibitor of angiogenesis. *Proc Natl Acad Sci USA* 1994;91:4082–5.
14. Kenyon BM, Browne F, D'Amato RJ. Effects of thalidomide and related metabolites in a mouse corneal model of neovascularization. *Exp Eye Res* 1997;64:971–8.
15. Kotoh T, Dhar DK, Masunaga R et al. Antiangiogenic therapy of human esophageal cancers with thalidomide in nude mice. *Surgery* 1999;125:536–44.
16. Ribatti D, Vacca A, De Falco G et al. Angiogenesis, angiogenic factor expression and hematological malignancies. *Anticancer Res* 2001;21:4333–9.
17. Vacca A, Ribatti D, Presta M et al. Bone marrow neovascularization, plasma cell angiogenic potential, and matrix metalloproteinase-2 secretion parallel progression of human multiple myeloma. *Blood* 1999;93:3064–73.
18. Singhal S, Mehta J, Desikan R et al. Antitumor activity of thalidomide in refractory multiple myeloma. *N Engl J Med* 1999;341:1565–71.
19. Barlogie B, Desikan R, Eddlemon P et al. Extended survival in advanced and refractory multiple myeloma after single-agent thalidomide: identification of prognostic factors in a phase 2 study of 169 patients. *Blood* 2001;98:492–4.
20. Stirling D. Thalidomide: a novel template for anticancer drugs. *Semin Oncol* 2001;28:602–6.
21. Mitsiades CS, Treon SP, Mitsiades N et al. TRAIL/Apo2L ligand selectively induces apoptosis and overcomes drug resistance in multiple myeloma: therapeutic applications. *Blood* 2001;98:795–804.
22. Mitsiades N, Mitsiades CS, Poulaki V et al. Apoptotic signaling induced by immunomodulatory thalidomide analogs in human multiple myeloma cells: therapeutic implications. *Blood* 2002;99:4525–30.
23. Hideshima T, Chauhan D, Shima Y et al. Thalidomide and its analogs overcome drug resistance of human multiple myeloma cells to conventional therapy. *Blood* 2000;96:2943–50.

24. Davies FE, Raje N, Hideshima T et al. Thalidomide and immunomodulatory derivatives augment natural killer cell cytotoxicity in multiple myeloma. *Blood* 2001;98:210–6.
25. Lentzsch S, Rogers MS, LeBlanc R et al. S-3-Amino-phthalimido-glutarimide inhibits angiogenesis and growth of B-cell neoplasias in mice. *Cancer Res* 2002;62:2300–5.
26. King RW, Deshaies RJ, Peters JM et al. How proteolysis drives the cell cycle. *Science* 1996;274:1652–9.
27. Kisselev AF, Goldberg AL. Proteasome inhibitors: from research tools to drug candidates. *Chem Biol* 2001;8:739–58.
28. Adams J, Palombella VJ, Sausville EA et al. Proteasome inhibitors: a novel class of potent and effective antitumor agents. *Cancer Res* 1999;59:2615–22.
29. Orlowski RZ, Eswara JR, Lafond-Walker A et al. Tumor growth inhibition induced in a murine model of human Burkitt's lymphoma by a proteasome inhibitor. *Cancer Res* 1998;58:4342–8.
30. Tan C, Waldmann TA. Proteasome inhibitor PS-341, a potential therapeutic agent for adult T-cell leukemia. *Cancer Res* 2002;62:1083–6.
31. Teicher BA, Ara G, Herbst R et al. The proteasome inhibitor PS-341 in cancer therapy. *Clin Cancer Res* 1999;5:2638–45.
32. Harbison MT, Bruns CJ, Bold RJ et al. Proteasome inhibitor PS-341 is effective as an anti-angiogenic agent in the treatment of human pancreatic carcinoma via the inhibition of NF-κB and subsequent inhibition of vascular endothelial growth factor production. *Proc Am Assoc Cancer Res* 2000;41:71.
33. Vescio RA, Cao J, Hong CH et al. Myeloma Ig heavy chain V region sequences reveal prior antigenic selection and marked somatic mutation but no intraclonal diversity. *J Immunol* 1995;155:2487–97.
34. Mitsiades N, Mitsiades CS, Poulaki V et al. Molecular sequelae of proteasome inhibition in human multiple myeloma cells. *Proc Natl Acad Sci USA* 2002;99:14374–9.
35. Hideshima T, Mitsiades C, Akiyama M et al. Molecular mechanisms mediating antimyeloma activity of proteasome inhibitor PS-341. *Blood* 2003;101:1530–4.
36. Mitsiades N, Mitsiades CS, Richardson PG et al. The proteasome inhibitor PS-341 potentiates sensitivity of multiple myeloma cells to conventional chemotherapeutic agents: therapeutic applications. *Blood* 2003;101:2377–80.
37. Orlowski RZ, Stinchcombe TE, Mitchell BS et al. Phase I trial of the proteasome inhibitor PS-341 in patients with refractory hematologic malignancies. *J Clin Oncol* 2002;20:4420–7.
38. Bladé J, Samson D, Reece D et al. Criteria for evaluating disease response and progression in patients with multiple myeloma treated by high-dose therapy and haemopoietic stem cell transplantation. Myeloma Subcommittee of the EBMT. European Group for Blood and Marrow Transplant. *Br J Haematol* 1998;102:1115–23.
39. Jagannath S, Barlogie B, Berenson J et al. A phase II multicenter randomized study of the proteasome inhibitor bortezomib (VELCADE, formerly PS-341) in multiple myeloma (MM) patients (pts) relapsed after front-line therapy. *Blood* 2002;100:812A (Abstr.).
40. Shao W, Fanelli M, Ferrara FF et al. Arsenic trioxide as an inducer of apoptosis and loss of PML/RAR alpha protein in acute promyelocytic leukemia cells. *J Natl Cancer Inst* 1998;90:124–133.
41. Rousselot P, Labaume S, Marolleau JP et al. Arsenic trioxide and melarsoprol induce apoptosis in plasma cell lines and in plasma cells from myeloma patients. *Cancer Res* 1999;59:1041–8.
42. Park WH, Seol JG, Kim ES et al. Arsenic trioxide-mediated growth inhibition in MC/CAR myeloma cells via cell cycle arrest in association with induction of cyclin-dependent kinase inhibitor, p21, and apoptosis. *Cancer Res* 2000;60:3065–71.

43. Hayashi T, Hideshima T, Akiyama M et al. Arsenic trioxide inhibits growth of human multiple myeloma cells in the bone marrow microenvironment. *Mol Cancer Ther* 2002;1:851–60.
44. Deaglio S, Canella D, Baj G et al. Evidence of an immunologic mechanism behind the therapeutical effects of arsenic trioxide (As_2O3) on myeloma cells. *Leuk Res* 2001;25:227–35.
45. Grad JM, Bahlis NJ, Reis I et al. Ascorbic acid enhances arsenic trioxide-induced cytotoxicity in multiple myeloma cells. *Blood* 2001;98:805–13.
46. Podar K, Tai YT, Davies FE et al. Vascular endothelial growth factor triggers signaling cascades mediating multiple myeloma cell growth and migration. *Blood* 2001;98:428–35.
47. Podar K, Tai YT, Lin BK et al. Vascular endothelial growth factor-induced migration of multiple myeloma cells is associated with beta 1 integrin- and phosphatidylinositol 3-kinase-dependent PKC alpha activation. *J Biol Chem* 2001;277:7875–81.
48. Bellamy WT, Richter L, Frutiger Y et al. Expression of vascular endothelial growth factor and its receptors in hematopoietic malignancies. *Cancer Res* 1999;59:728–33.
49. Dankbar B, Padro T, Leo R et al. Vascular endothelial growth factor and interleukin-6 in paracrine tumor-stromal cell interactions in multiple myeloma. *Blood* 2000;95:2630–6.
50. Gupta D, Treon SP, Shima Y et al. Adherence of multiple myeloma cells to bone marrow stromal cells upregulates vascular endothelial growth factor secretion: therapeutic applications. *Leukemia* 2001;15:1950–61.
51. Lin B, Podar K, Gupta D et al. The vascular endothelial growth factor receptor kinase inhibitor PTK787/ZK222584 inhibits growth and migration of multiple myeloma cells in the bone marrow microenvironment. *Cancer Res* 2002;62:5019–26.
52. Mitsiades N, Mitsiades CS, Poulaki V et al. Intracellular regulation of tumor necrosis factor-related apoptosis-inducing ligand-induced apoptosis in human multiple myeloma cells. *Blood* 2002;99:2162–71.
53. D'Amato RJ, Lin CM, Flynn E et al. 2-Methoxyestradiol, an endogenous mammalian metabolite, inhibits tubulin polymerization by interacting at the colchicine site. *Proc Natl Acad Sci USA* 1994;91:3964–8.
54. Klauber N, Parangi S, Flynn E et al. Inhibition of angiogenesis and breast cancer in mice by the microtubule inhibitors 2-methoxyestradiol and taxol. *Cancer Res* 1997;57:81–6.
55. Chauhan D, Li G, Auclair D et al. Identification of genes regulated by 2-Methoxyestradiol (2ME2) in multiple myeloma (MM) cells using oligonucleotides arrays. *Blood* 2003;101:3606–14.
56. Chauhan D, Catley L, Hideshima T et al. 2-Methoxyestradiol overcomes drug resistance in multiple myeloma cells. *Blood* 2002;100:2187–94.
57. Kato K, Cox AD, Hisaka MM et al. Isoprenoid addition to Ras protein is the critical modification for its membrane association and transforming activity. *Proc Natl Acad Sci USA* 1992;89:6403–7.
58. Karp JE, Kaufmann SH, Adjei AA et al. Current status of clinical trials of farnesyltransferase inhibitors. *Curr Opin Oncol* 2001;13:470–6.
59. Mitsiades CS, Mitsiades N, Poulaki V et al. Activation of NF-kappaB and upregulation of intracellular anti-apoptotic proteins via the IGF-1/Akt signaling in human multiple myeloma cells: therapeutic implications. *Oncogene* 2002;21:5673–83.
60. Adjei AA, Davis JN, Bruzek LM et al. Synergy of the protein farnesyltransferase inhibitor SCH66336 and cisplatin in human cancer cell lines. *Clin Cancer Res* 2001;7:1438–45.
61. Karp JE, Lancet JE, Kaufmann SH et al. Clinical and biologic activity of the farnesyltransferase inhibitor R115777 in adults with refractory and relapsed acute leukemias: a phase 1 clinical-laboratory correlative trial. *Blood* 2001;97:3361–9.

62. Mitsiades N, Mitsiades CS, Richardson PG et al. Molecular sequelae of histone deacetylase inhibition in human malignant B cells. *Blood* 2003;101:4055–62.
63. Mauro MJ, O'Dwyer M, Heinrich MC et al. STI571: a paradigm of new agents for cancer therapeutics. *J Clin Oncol* 2002;20:325–34.
64. Jing Y, Xia L, Waxman S. Targeted removal of PML-RARalpha protein is required prior to inhibition of histone deacetylase for overcoming all-trans retinoic acid differentiation resistance in acute promyelocytic leukemia. *Blood* 2002;100:1008–13.

4

Thalidomide treatment

Donna M Weber

Introduction

Multiple myeloma (MM) is a proliferation of malignant plasma cells that produces a monoclonal (M) immunoglobulin. This disseminated malignancy is diagnosed in approximately 14,500 Americans each year, and, though treatable, accounts for 2% of all cancer deaths and remains incurable. Treatment can be deferred in around 20% of patients without symptoms, but all patients eventually require chemotherapy.

For many years, intermittent courses of melphalan and prednisone have constituted the standard therapy for newly diagnosed patients with symptomatic MM. Many other drug combinations have been studied, including combinations of alkylating agents, vincristine, and anthracyclines, but there has been no consistent survival gain over melphalan and prednisone [1]. High-dose dexamethasone regimens (including vincristine, doxorubicin, and dexamethasone [VAD] chemotherapy) induce rapid responses, and have resulted in improved survival for many patients when followed by intensive therapy with autologous stem cell support early in the disease course [2]. However, all MM patients eventually relapse, and with increased resistance to retreatment. This accounts for the current median survival time of approximately 4 years for symptomatic patients.

The antiangiogenic properties of thalidomide *in vitro*, and the increased vascularization of bone marrow in patients with advanced MM, resulted in assessment of this drug at the

University of Arkansas in patients with advanced, resistant MM [3–5]. Out of five initial patients in this pilot study, one achieved near complete remission (CR), prompting a Phase II trial of thalidomide [3]. This confirmed an approximate 25% partial remission (PR) rate when standard criteria of 50% serum paraprotein reduction are considered [6]. Such clinical activity has been confirmed by others (see **Table 1**). This chapter focuses on the results of recent clinical trials with thalidomide in MM.

Pharmacology

Thalidomide was initially used as a sedative. In the 1950s it was also found to be effective for the treatment of morning sickness. It was withdrawn in the early 1960s due to frequent teratogenicity (phocomelia) [7]. Thalidomide is a glutamic acid derivative that consists of a chiral center and two amide rings. It is categorized as an immunomodulatory agent, and has antiangiogenic properties *in vitro* [8,9]. At physiologic pH, thalidomide exists as a racemic mixture; while the S-isomer appears to be responsible for teratogenicity, the R-isomer results in sedation. These isomers interconvert, making attempts at separating the R-isomer unsuccessful [9].

Due to thalidomide's insolubility in water, an intravenous preparation is not currently available. The drug's pharmacokinetics have not been well characterized, and appear to vary among patients. Following administration of 200 mg thalidomide, maximum serum concentration is reached within an average of 4 hours; the drug undergoes spontaneous, nonenzymatic, hydrolytic cleavage to numerous metabolites, which are rapidly excreted in urine, while unabsorbed drug is excreted in feces. For a 200 mg dose of thalidomide, the mean half-life in blood ranges from 4–9 hours, while doses of 800 mg have a longer half-life of approximately 8 hours [9–11]. Although the appropriate dose adjustments for patients with renal and hepatic failure have not been well established, moderate doses have been tolerated in patients with renal failure.

Study	Daily thalidomide dose (mg)
Single-agent trials	
Singhal et al. [6]	200–800
Weber et al. [23,24]	100–400
Durie et al. [25]	50–400
Juliusson et al. [41]	200–800
Rajkumar et al. [44]	200–800
Raza et al. [45]	200–800
Tosi et al. [46]	100–800
Yakoub-Agha et al. [47]	50–800
Barlogie et al. [22]	200–800
Grosbois et al. [48]	200–800
Hus et al. [49]	200–400
Combination trials	
Weber et al. [23,38]	200–800 + dexamethasone
Coleman et al. [26]	50–200 + clarithromycin, dexamethasone
Kropff et al. [50]	100–400 + dexamethasone
Barlogie et al. [33]	400 + dexamethasone, cisplatin, doxorubicin, cyclophosphamide, etoposide
Dimopoulos et al. [32]	200–800 + dexamethasone
Moehler et al. [51]	400 + cyclophosphamide, etoposide, dexamethasone
Palumbo et al. [52]	100 + dexamethasone
Tosi et al. [53]	100 + dexamethasone

Table 1. Results from clinical trials of thalidomide in patients with resistant multiple myeloma. Response to treatment was defined by ≥50% reduction in monoclonal protein levels.

Thalidomide has demonstrated apoptotic, immunomodulatory, and antiangiogenic effects *in vitro*. The antiangiogenic effects may arise from metabolites that interrupt angiogenesis, mediated by basic fibroblast growth factor (bFGF) and/or vascular endothelial growth factor (VEGF) [3,12,13]. In addition, thalidomide inhibits tumor necrosis factor (TNF)-α gene activation by decreasing nuclear factor-κB binding [14]. Despite the correlation between marrow angiogenesis factors and disease activity in MM, and between increased levels of angiogenic cytokines (bFGF and VEGF) and an advanced disease state, no correlation has been established between increased microvascular density and posttreatment decline in neovascularization in patients with disease responding to thalidomide [4–6,13,15,16]. Inhibition of angiogenesis alone is unlikely to account for the therapeutic effect of thalidomide against MM.

Thalidomide and its analogues directly inhibit the growth of plasma cells *in vitro*, possibly via caspase-8 activation and subsequent apoptosis [10,17]. TNF-α stimulates bone marrow stromal cell (BMSC) secretion of interleukin (IL)-6, and induces the expression of adhesion molecules (lymphocyte function-associated antigen-1, intercellular adhesion molecule-1, and vascular cell adhesion molecule-1) on MM cells and BMSCs [10,18]. Since thalidomide inhibits TNF-α, expression of these adhesion molecules on BMSCs may be decreased by treatment, resulting in inhibition of MM cell adhesion and reduction of TNF-α-stimulated IL-6 secretion [19]. Thalidomide may also promote the growth of stimulated anti-CD3 T cells, which might increase levels of cytokines (interferon [IFN]-α or IL-12) that inhibit MM cell growth [20].

While the mechanism for the antimyeloma effect of thalidomide remains unclear, there is a clear apoptotic effect *in vitro* that is enhanced by dexamethasone. This combined effect can be overcome by IL-6, which is consistent with IL-6 suppression being a contributing factor to the antimyeloma effect of thalidomide [21].

Dose

The optimum dose of thalidomide for MM patients (they are often older and more debilitated than patients with other cancers) has not been formally evaluated in a Phase I trial. At the University of Arkansas, patients who received ≥42 g of thalidomide over 3 months (approximately 400 mg/d) had a higher frequency of response (54%) and higher 2-year survival rate (63%) than comparable patients who received <42 g (21% and 45%, respectively; $P<0.001$) [22]. The median cumulative dose of 42 g was not defined as a continuous variable, which may have provided a different result.

At the University of Texas MD Anderson Cancer Center, the response rate with doses ≤400 mg/d was similar to that seen with higher doses, but with fewer side effects [23,24]. Other studies have reported responses at doses of ≤100 mg/d [25,26], but no systematic evaluation has been made, so recommendations for dosing remain difficult and empiric.

Toxicity

Thalidomide is teratogenic and is absolutely contraindicated in pregnant women. All patients treated in the US must be registered on the System for Thalidomide Education and Prescribing Safety (STEPS) program before thalidomide may be prescribed and dispensed [27]. Women of childbearing potential (premenopausal and <2 years postmenopausal) who are prescribed thalidomide are required to take a pregnancy test, continue on two effective forms of birth control, and have further pregnancy tests every 4 weeks. Men receiving thalidomide must either abstain from sex or use a latex condom.

Since sedation is a frequent side effect, thalidomide should be taken at bedtime, though fatigue may be a problem on the following day [6,10,23,24,28]. Constipation – another common side effect – should be prevented and controlled by a combination of generous fluid intake, stool softeners, and laxatives [6,10,23,24,28]. Dry skin and pruritis are frequent, but can often be prevented by nonalcohol-based lubricants and the avoidance of hot baths. An erythematous macular skin rash may occur that requires cessation of thalidomide until clearing, with resumption at a lower dose. Rarely, cases of Stevens–Johnson syndrome have been reported in patients treated with thalidomide and concurrent dexamethasone [28]. A sensorimotor peripheral neuropathy, usually of the feet, may be a problem, particularly after prolonged exposure to thalidomide [10,24,28]. Less commonly, peripheral edema, tremors, bradycardia, hypothyroidism, and, rarely, neutropenia and hepatic enzyme elevation have been observed [6,10,23,24,28].

While thrombotic and embolic events are uncommon with single-agent thalidomide (in our experience) [29], the incidence is higher (~15%) when thalidomide is combined with either steroids or a steroid–anthracycline combination [30,31]. Among 24 previously untreated patients given thalidomide and dexamethasone, despite prophylactic warfarin (1 mg orally, every day) we noted six thrombotic episodes. Subsequent therapeutic anticoagulation in all patients has virtually eliminated this problem, though this approach must consider the risk of bleeding, particularly for those at risk of ulcers and gastrointestinal bleeding with added dexamethasone. Therapeutic anticoagulation should be strongly considered in those patients with other risk factors that place them at higher risk for thrombosis. Further research is necessary to clarify the role of either prophylactic or therapeutic anticoagulation in myeloma patients receiving treatment with thalidomide and dexamethasone.

Clinical trials

Refractory disease

Single-agent thalidomide

Singhal et al. published results of a Phase II trial of thalidomide involving 84 patients with advanced refractory MM, of whom

76 had previously received myeloablative therapy with stem cell support [6]. Patients received 200 mg/d thalidomide with a dose escalation of 200 mg increments every 2 weeks – in the absence of side effects – to a maximum of 800 mg/d. The median duration of treatment was 80 days. Twenty-one patients (25%) achieved PR based on >50% reduction in serum M protein [6]. In a recent update of this study, 30% of 169 patients responded by these same criteria [22]. The 2-year event-free and overall survival rates were 20% and 48%, respectively, in these patients with advanced MM, with higher 2-year survival rates among responsive versus unresponsive patients (69% and 47%, respectively; $P = 0.01$). Higher event-free survival rates were observed in patients with normal cytogenetics, a low plasma cell labeling index, and β_2-microglobulin levels <3 mg/L [22]. Using similar criteria, Weber and coworkers confirmed a response rate of 25% and projected median remission duration of 15 months in a Phase II study of 44 evaluable patients with resistant disease [23,24].

Many other trials have confirmed the approximately 25% response rate of single-agent thalidomide in refractory MM (see **Table 1**). Some of these trials used less-stringent criteria for defining remission – stable disease or only 25% reduction in M protein levels – whereas most centers applied the historical standard of ≥50% reduction in M paraprotein.

Thalidomide in combination with other agents

In 1999, a trial of thalidomide (at doses similar to those noted above for single-agent use) with intermittent dexamethasone (20 mg/m^2/d orally on days 1–5 and 15–19, repeated around day 30 for a total of two courses, followed by maintenance on days 1–5 only every 4 weeks) was performed [23,28]. Among 47 patients with resistant MM, 46% achieved remission despite prior resistance to both thalidomide and high-dose intermittent dexamethasone administered as single agents. In view of this, the effects of thalidomide and dexamethasone appear to be synergistic. A similar response rate of 55% was observed by Dimopoulos et al. in 44 patients with refractory MM [32].

Investigators at the University of Arkansas are evaluating a program of dexamethasone, cyclophosphamide, etoposide, and cisplatin (DCEP) in combination with thalidomide, comparing it with DCEP alone, in patients with relapsing high tumor mass disease or with poor prognostic cytogenetics [33]. After a median follow-up period of 17 months, the response rate of 18% (after 3 cycles of DCEP) doubled to 36% with the addition of thalidomide.

The same group has studied the DT-PACE regimen (dexamethasone, thalidomide, cisplatin, doxorubicin, cyclophosphamide, and etoposide) in patients with prior therapy versus intensive therapy with autologous stem cell transplantation [33]. Among the first 179 patients treated with DT-PACE, only 45% (80 patients) were randomized to the study, largely due to low frequency of response [33]. CR was noted in 26 of 39 patients who received tandem transplants, but in only 11 of 41 patients continuing on DT-PACE ($P<0.01$). Two-year event-free survival rates were similar (73%) in both groups, but 33 patients who failed DT-PACE received later tandem transplants, making the result difficult to interpret. Due to the inferior results with continued DT-PACE, the study has been amended to include melphalan (100 mg/m^2) with peripheral blood stem cell support in the DT-PACE arm.

A study of VAD [30] combined with thalidomide in refractory patients was terminated prematurely because of a high rate of thrombotic complications, which were attributed to the combination of doxorubicin and dexamethasone. Combination studies are summarized in **Table 1**.

Previously untreated disease

Single-agent thalidomide

Because thalidomide was effective in the treatment of patients with refractory MM, several groups have used this drug in patients with previously untreated MM. Since the efficacy of thalidomide as a single agent has not been defined, we evaluated thalidomide 100–200 mg/m^2/d, escalating to 400 mg/m^2/d, in patients with asymptomatic MM [34]. Twenty-eight patients considered to be at high risk for early progression of disease, as determined by criteria previously established, were included. PR, defined as ≥75% reduction in serum myeloma protein synthesis and/or ≥95% reduction in Bence Jones protein, was noted in 36% of patients.

In a similar trial that was initiated in 1999 and has recently been updated, Rajkumar et al. found a comparable response rate of 34% among 29 patients [35–37]. The value of long-term therapy remains unclear in terms of delaying the time to progression before the need for conventional chemotherapy, or producing an effect on survival: this requires many years of study in view of the long period of stability of asymptomatic disease. Since early treatment of the asymptomatic patient with other agents has not previously improved survival, the value of thalidomide in asymptomatic disease should be restricted to clinical trials until the benefits and long-term side effects are established.

Thalidomide in combination with other agents

The activity of thalidomide with dexamethasone in patients with refractory disease stimulated further trials of this regimen in previously untreated patients with symptomatic disease. Rajkumar et al. reported on 50 patients treated with thalidomide (200 mg/d with a dose escalation of 200 mg/d every 2 weeks up to 800 mg/d) combined with dexamethasone (40 mg/d on days 1–4, 9–12, and 17–20 on odd cycles [28-days], and days 1–4 on even cycles) [28]. Two of the first seven patients experienced grade 3–4 skin toxicity, which resulted in subsequent patients receiving a constant dose of 200 mg/d. Thirty-two patients (64%) showed ≥50% reduction of serum M protein. Stem cell harvest was completed without difficulty in 31 patients, and 26 patients proceeded to myeloablative therapy with stem cell support.

In a similar trial at the University of Texas MD Anderson Cancer Center, 40 previously untreated MM patients were given 100–200 mg thalidomide at bedtime, with dose escalations as

Disease status	Study	Year	Daily thalidomide dose (mg)	*N*	Response rate (%)
Asymptomatic	Weber et al. [29,34]	2000, 2003	100–400	28	36
	Rajkumar et al. [35–37]	2000, 2001, 2003	200–800	16	38
Symptomatic	Rajkumar et al. [28,54]	2001, 2002	200–400[1] + Dex	50	64
	Weber et al. [29,38]	2001, 2003	100–400 + Dex	40	72

Table 2. Results from clinical trials of thalidomide in previously untreated multiple myeloma patients. Response to treatment was defined by ≥50% reduction in monoclonal protein levels. Dex: dexamethasone. [1]Because two of seven initial patients experienced grade 3–4 skin toxicity, subsequent patients received a fixed dose of 200 mg daily.

tolerated up to 400 mg [38]. Dexamethasone (20 mg/m^2/d) was given on days 1–4, 9–12, and 17–20 for two 28-day courses, followed by dexamethasone on days 1–4 (repeated on approx. day 28) for maintenance only until relapse. Twenty-nine patients showed ≥75% reduction in serum M protein synthesis and/or ≥95% reduction in Bence Jones proteinuria, achieving a response rate of 72%; CR was noted in seven patients (18%). Successful stem cell harvest was possible for all responding patients when attempted. Results from recent trials in previously untreated MM patients are summarized in **Table 2.**

Consolidation and maintenance therapy after intensive therapy with stem cell support

CR correlates with increased survival in patients with MM [39]. In order to convert PR to CR, Alexanian et al. treated 21 patients with thalidomide and dexamethasone after stability was achieved with myeloablative therapy in addition to stem cell support [40]. Combined thalidomide and dexamethasone was given within

15 months of intensive therapy. Thalidomide was initiated at a daily dose of 100 mg and escalated to a maximum dose of 300 mg. A dexamethasone dose of 20 mg/m^2 was given on days 1–4, 9–12, and 17–20, with resumption of the same schedule on approximately day 30 (dexamethasone administration was subsequently decreased to days 1–4 only each month). Fifty-seven percent of patients demonstrated a further marked reduction (≥90%) of M protein levels, including four patients whose PR was converted to CR [40]. Further controlled trials are required to determine whether such an effect may produce longer periods of disease-free survival.

Extramedullary extension of bone plasmacytoma or extramedullary plasmacytoma

Although thalidomide given either alone or in combination is effective against both untreated and resistant MM, its success in patients with extramedullary plasmacytoma appears less encouraging. Juliusson et al. described one patient who showed a rapid response of monoclonal immunoglobulin (Ig)A, but developed paraparesis due to progression of a spinal plasmacytoma [41]. The authors hypothesized that differences in microvascular supply of marrow and the extramedullary tumor might explain the different effects. Similarly, Bladé et al. described the resistance of extramedullary plasmacytomas in five patients despite reduction of paraprotein in three patients [42]. Myers et al. also reported lack of response in extraosseous disease of two patients treated with thalidomide, despite reduction of M IgAλ [43].

At the University of Texas MD Anderson Cancer Center, progression of a paraspinal mass after treatment with combined thalidomide and dexamethasone was also noted, despite a marked reduction in IgAλ paraprotein levels. In contrast, at the same institution we have observed the reduction of an extramedullary extension of a rib lesion and IgGκ paraprotein in one patient treated for resistant MM. The biologic and prognostic significance and sensitivity of extramedullary disease and/or IgAλ paraprotein during thalidomide treatment requires clarification in future trials.

Conclusions

Thalidomide is an effective agent in the treatment of patients with either resistant or previously untreated MM. Although thalidomide is active, side effects such as constipation, fatigue, neuropathy, and thrombotic/embolic complications may limit its use in some patients. Newer nonteratogenic derivatives – such as the IMiDs (immunomodulatory thalidomide analogs) – are also effective, but have a different spectrum of side effects, and clinical experience with them remains limited [55,56]. Combinations of these new agents (thalidomide, IMiDs, proteasome inhibitors, dexamethasone) followed by early intensive therapy with stem cell support may result in higher response rates with more CRs, longer unmaintained or maintained remissions, and improved survival rates for more patients.

Acknowledgements

The author has received thalidomide from Celgene Corporation for clinical research into MM. The author is indebted to Raymond Alexanian, MD, for his mentorship and editorial assistance with this chapter.

References

1. Myeloma Trialist's Collaborative Group. Combination chemotherapy versus melphalan plus prednisone as treatment for multiple myeloma: an overview of 6,633 patients from 27 randomized trials. *J Clin Oncol* 1998;16:3832–42.
2. Barlogie B, Smith L, Alexanian R. Effective treatment of advanced myeloma refractory to alkylating agents. *N Engl J Med* 1984;310:1353–6.
3. D'Amato RJ, Loughnan MS, Flynn E et al. Thalidomide is an inhibitor of angiogenesis. *Proc Natl Acad Sci USA* 1994;91:4082–5.
4. Vacca A, Ribatti D, Roncali L et al. Bone marrow angiogenesis and progression in multiple myeloma. *Br J Hematol* 1994;87:503–8.
5. Munshi N, Wilson CS, Penn J et al. Angiogenesis in newly diagnosed multiple myeloma: poor prognosis with increased microvessel density (MVD) in bone marrow biopsies. *Blood* 1998;92(Suppl. 2):98A (Abstr.)
6. Singhal S, Mehta J, Desikan R. Antitumor activity of thalidomide in refractory multiple myeloma [published erratum appears in *N Engl J Med* 2000;342:364]. *N Engl J Med* 1999;341:1565–71.
7. Lenz W. Thalidomide and congenital abnormalities. *Lancet* 1962;1:45.

8. Tsengs S, Pak G, Washenik K et al. Rediscovering thalidomide: a review of its mechanism of action, side effects, and potential uses. *J Am Acad Dermatol* 1996;35:969–79.
9. Stirling DL. Pharmacology of thalidomide. *Semin Hematol* 2000;37(1 Suppl. 3):5–14.
10. Richardson P, Hideshima T, Anderson K. Thalidomide: emerging role in cancer medicine. *Annu Rev Med* 2002;53:629–57.
11. Chen TL, Vogelsang GB, Petty BG et al. Plasma pharmacokinetics and urinary excretion of thalidomide after oral dosing in healthy male volunteers. *Drug Metab Dispos* 1989;17:402–5.
12. Kenyon BM, Browne F, D'Amato RJ. Effects of thalidomide and related metabolites in a mouse corneal model of neovascularization. *Exp Eye Res* 1997;64:971–8.
13. Podor K, Tai Y-T, Davies FE et al. Vascular endothelial growth factor triggers signaling cascades mediating multiple myeloma cell growth and migration. *Blood* 2001;98:428–35.
14. Turk BE, Jiang H, Liu JO. Binding of thalidomide to α1-acid glycoprotein may be involved in its inhibition of tumor necrosis factor-α production. *Proc Natl Acad Sci USA* 1996;93:7552–6.
15. Vacca A, Ribatti D, Presta M et al. Bone marrow neovascularization, plasma cell angiogenic potential, and matrix metalloproteinase-2 secretion parallel progression of human multiple myeloma. *Blood* 1999;93:3064–73.
16. Bellamy WT, Richter L, Frutiger Y et al. Expression of vascular endothelial growth factor and its receptor in hematopoietic malignancies. *Cancer Res* 1999;59:728–33.
17. Mitsiades N, Mitsiades CS, Poulaki V et al. Apoptotic signaling induced by immunomodulatory thalidomide analogs (IMiDs) in human multiple myeloma cells: therapeutic implications. *Blood* 2001;98:775A (Abstr.).
18. Witzig TE. The role of adhesion receptors in the pathogenesis of multiple myeloma. *Hematol Oncol Clin North Am* 1999;13:1127–43.
19. Sampio EP, Sarno EN, Galilly R et al. Thalidomide selectively inhibits tumor necrosis factor alpha production by stimulated human monocytes. *J Exp Med* 1991;173:699–703.
20. Davies FE, Raje N, Hideshima T et al. Thalidomide and immunomodulatory derivatives augment natural killer cell cytotoxicity in multiple myeloma. *Blood* 2001;98:210–6.
21. Hideshima T, Chauhan D, Shima Y et al. Thalidomide and its analogs overcome drug resistance of human multiple myeloma cells to conventional therapy. *Blood* 2000;96:2943–50.
22. Barlogie B, Desikan R, Eddelmon P et al. Extended survival in advanced and refractory multiple myeloma after single-agent thalidomide: identification of prognostic factors in a phase 2 study of 169 patients. *Blood* 2001;98:492–4.
23. Weber DM, Gavino M, Delasalle K et al. Thalidomide alone or with dexamethasone for multiple myeloma. *Blood* 1999;94(Suppl. 1):604A (Abstr.).
24. Alexanian R, Weber D. Thalidomide for resistant and relapsing myeloma. *Semin Hematol* 2000;37(1 Suppl. 3):22S–25S.
25. Durie BGM, Stephan DE. Efficacy of low dose thalidomide (T) in multiple myeloma. *Blood* 1999;94(Suppl. 1):316A (Abstr.).
26. Coleman M, Leonard JP, Nahum K et al. Non-myelosuppressive therapy with BLT-D (Biaxin®, low dose thalidomide and dexamethasone) is highly active in Waldenstrom's macroglobulinemia and myeloma. *Blood* 2000;96:167A (Abstr.).
27. Zeldis JB, Williams BA, Thomas SD et al. S.T.E.P.S.: a comprehensive program for controlling and monitoring access to thalidomide. *Clin Ther* 1999;21:319–30.
28. Rajkumar SV, Dispenzieri A, Fonseca R et al. Thalidomide for previously untreated indolent or smoldering multiple myeloma. *Leukemia* 2001;15:1274–6.

29. Weber D, Rankin K, Gavino M et al. Thalidomide alone or with dexamethasone for previously untreated multiple myeloma. *J Clin Oncol* 2003;21:16–9.
30. Osman K, Comenzo R, Rajkumar SV. Deep venous thrombosis and thalidomide therapy for multiple myeloma. *N Engl J Med* 2001;344:1951–2.
31. Zangari M, Siegel E, Barlogie B et al. Thrombogenic activity of doxorubicin in myeloma patients receiving thalidomide: implications for therapy. *Blood* 2002;100:1168–71.
32. Dimopoulos MA, Zervas K, Kouvatseas G et al. Thalidomide and dexamethasone combination for refractory multiple myeloma. *Ann Oncol* 2001;12:991–5.
33. Barlogie B, Zangari M, Spencer T et al. Thalidomide in the management of multiple myeloma. *Semin Hematol* 2001;38:250–9.
34. Weber DM, Rankin K, Gavino M et al. Angiogenesis factors and sensitivity to thalidomide in previously untreated multiple myeloma (MM). *Blood* 2000;96:168A.
35. Rajkumar SV, Hayman S, Fonseca R et al. Thalidomide plus dexamethasone (Thal/dex) and thalidomide alone (Thal) as first line therapy for newly diagnosed myeloma (MM). *Blood* 2000;96:168A (Abstr.).
36. Rajkumar SV, Hayman SR, Gertz MA et al. Combination therapy with thalidomide plus dexamethasone (Thal/dex) for newly diagnosed myeloma (MM). *Blood* 2001;98:849A (Abstr.).
37. Rajkumar SV, Gertz MA, Lacy MQ et al. Thalidomide as initial therapy for early-stage myeloma. *Leukemia* 2003;17:775–9.
38. Weber DM, Rankin K, Delasalle K et al. Thalidomide alone and in combination for previously untreated myeloma. Program and abstracts of the VIII International Myeloma Workshop; 2001 May 4–8; Banff, Alta., Canada. S66 (Abstr.).
39. Alexanian R, Weber D, Giralt S et al. Impact of complete remission with intensive therapy in patients with responsive multiple myeloma. *Bone Marrow Transplant* 2001;27:1037–43.
40. Alexanian R, Weber D, Giralt S et al. Consolidation therapy of multiple myeloma with thalidomide-dexamethasone after intensive chemotherapy. *Ann Oncol* 2002;13:1116–9.
41. Juliusson G, Celsing F, Turesson I et al. Frequent good partial remissions from thalidomide including best response ever in patients with advanced refractory and relapsed myeloma. *Br J Haematol* 2000;109:89–96.
42. Blade J, Perales M, Rosinol L et al. Thalidomide in multiple myeloma: lack of response of soft-tissue plasmacytomas. *Br J Hematol* 2001;113:422–4.
43. Myers B, Grimley C, Crouch D et al. Lack of response to thalidomide in plasmacytomas. *Br J Haematol* 2001;115–234.
44. Rajkumar SV, Fonseca R, Dispenzieri A et al. A phase II trial of thalidomide in the treatment of relapsed multiple myeloma (MM) with laboratory correlative studies. *Blood* 2000;96:168A (Abstr.).
45. Raza SN, Veklser Y, Sabir T et al. Durable response to thalidomide in relapsed/refractory multiple myeloma. *Blood* 2000;96:168A (Abstr.).
46. Tosi P, Ronconi S, Zamagni E et al. Salvage therapy with thalidomide for patients with advanced relapsed/refractory multiple myeloma. *Blood* 2000;96:296b (Abstr.).
47. Yakoub-Agha I, Attal M, Dumontet C et al. Thalidomide in patients with advanced multiple myeloma: survival prognostic factors. *Blood* 2000;96:167A (Abstr.).
48. Grosbois B, Bellissant E, Moreau P et al. Thalidomide (thal) in the treatment of advanced multiple myeloma (MM). A prospective study of 120 patients. *Blood* 2001:98(Suppl. 1):163A (Abstr.).
49. Hus M, Dmoszynska A, Soroka-Wojtaszko M et al. Thalidomide treatment of resistant or relapsed multiple myeloma patients. *Haematologica* 2001;86:404–8.

50. Kropff MH, Innig G, Mitterer M et al. Hyperfractionated cyclophosphamide in combination with pulsed dexamethasone and thalidomide (Hyper-CDT) in primary refractory or relapsed multiple myeloma. *Blood* 2000;96:168A (Abstr.).
51. Moehler TM, Neben K, Benner A et al. Salvage therapy for multiple myeloma with thalidomide and CED chemotherapy. *Blood* 2001;98:3846–8.
52. Palumbo A, Giaccone L, Bertola A et al. Low-dose thalidomide plus dexamethasone is an effective salvage therapy for advanced myeloma. *Haematologica* 2001;86:399–403.
53 Tosi P, Zamagni E, Cellini C et al. Rapid response and early relapse after thalidomide plus dexamethasone salvage therapy in patients with advanced relapsed and refractory multiple myeloma. *Blood* 2001;98:163A (Abstr.).
54. Rajkumar SV, Hayman S, Gertz MA et al. Combination therapy with thalidomide plus dexamethasone for newly diagnosed myeloma. *J Clin Oncol* 2002;20:4319–23.
55. Richardson PG, Schlossman RL, Weller E et al. Immunomodulatory drug CC-5013 overcomes drug resistance and is well tolerated in patients with relapsed multiple myeloma. *Blood* 2002;100:3063–7.
56. Richardson PG, Jagannath S, Schlossman RL et al. A multi-center, randomized, phase II study to evaluate the efficacy and safety of two CDC-5013 dose regimens when used alone or in combination with dexamethasone for the treatment of relapsed or refractory multiple myeloma. *Blood* 2002;100:104a (Abstr. 386).

5

High-dose chemotherapy and bone marrow transplantation

Nikhil C Munshi, Robert L Schlossman, & Sundar Jagannath

Introduction

Multiple myeloma (MM) is the second most common hematologic malignancy. Left untreated, the median life expectancy of MM patients is <1 year. The introduction of alkylating agents and glucocorticoids in the 1960s offered effective palliation of the disease, with resolution of symptoms and signs of the disease, tumor regression lasting for a median of 18 months, and extension of the median life expectancy of MM patients beyond 30 months [1].

Over the next three decades, additional chemotherapeutic drugs were introduced for the management of MM, to be used either alone or in combination. Non-cross resistant drug combinations were evaluated for induction, as were chemotherapy or interferon (IFN) as maintenance strategies. While individual approaches appeared to improve treatment response rate and duration of remission, the median overall life expectancy of MM patients remained unchanged.

In the early 1980s, McElwain and Powles first reported that high doses of intravenous melphalan were able to overcome relative drug resistance and induce complete remission (CR) in previously treated MM patients [2]. While the duration and severity of myelosuppression was discouraging, it could be safely overcome with bone marrow (BM) and, later, stem cell rescue. Long-term follow-up of a number of clinical trials, both multicenter randomized studies as well as large single-center studies, has clearly shown the clinical utility of this approach in achieving CR and improving overall life expectancy. This chapter reviews the results of these studies and the role of stem cell transplantation (SCT) in MM.

Chemotherapy dose intensity

There is a log-linear dose–response effect in killing tumor cells *in vitro* with most alkylating agents [3]. However, translation of this into a clinically useful approach has been limited by the extramedullary toxicity of individual drugs. Therefore, dose escalation in a clinical setting is seldom >1 log (often 4–8 multiples) of the normal dose. This level of dose escalation has not been particularly helpful in overcoming drug resistance in solid tumors or refractory hematologic malignancies. However, in MM, McElwain reported that prior exposure or failure to respond to melphalan at a standard dose did not preclude subsequent induction of CR at higher doses [2]. Many other investigators have confirmed this observation [4–11].

Barlogie et al. reported the dose–response effect of melphalan in refractory MM [12]. Melphalan is a bifunctional alkylating agent with myelosuppression as its major toxicity. It is rapidly hydrolyzed into an inactive form in the plasma, with an elimination half-life ($t_{1/2}$ β) of 30–120 minutes; therefore, it is not dependent on kidney function for its elimination. This short half-life allows safe BM or stem cell infusion within 24 hours following melphalan; and high-dose melphalan can be administered to patients with impaired renal function [13]. As the dose is escalated from the standard 40 mg/m^2 to 70 mg/m^2 and 100 mg/m^2, the degree and duration of myelosuppression warrants growth factor support. Beyond 100 mg/m^2, stem cell rescue is required to keep treatment-related mortality <5% [14]. However, there is wide inter- and intrapatient pharmacokinetic variability, often >10-fold, even when melphalan is administered intravenously. The most frequent extramedullary toxicity encountered is gastrointestinal (GI), which is more often noted in the elderly and in patients with renal impairment. There have been occasional reports of unpredictable toxicity to the lung and veno-occlusive disease of the liver, especially when melphalan is combined with other agents, such as busulfan or carmustine.

For single-agent use, the dose of melphalan has been escalated to 200 mg/m^2 with blood progenitor cell support, and has been widely applied in tandem transplants with transplant-related mortality <5% [15]. In a select group of patients, the dose of melphalan has been further escalated (220–240 mg/m^2) with mucositis and GI toxicity being the predominant dose-limiting toxicities [16].

Other investigators have added total body irradiation (TBI) to melphalan to increase the dose intensity of the single agent [7,17,18]. At a melphalan does of 140 mg/m^2, the addition of TBI substantially improves tumor cytoreduction. However, the additive effect of TBI on GI toxicity limits the melphalan dose to a maximum of 140 mg/m^2. Dose escalation of melphalan to 160 mg/m^2, in combination with fractionated TBI of 12 Gy and infusional etoposide of 60 mg/kg, was given as intensification therapy to 100 MM patients in partial remission (PR) [19]. The treatment-related mortality rate was 12%, and was predominantly due to interstitial pneumonia, which affected 28% of patients.

Data from retrospective studies – both single-center [20] and the European Group for Blood and Marrow Transplantation (EBMT) Registry – show that patients receiving a regimen containing TBI fared poorly compared with those receiving melphalan alone [7,20]. This possibility was formally tested in a randomized study by the Intergroupe Francophone du Myelome (IFM), which compared melphalan (200 mg/m^2) with melphalan (140 mg/m^2) and TBI (8 Gy) in 282 newly diagnosed patients [21]. The response rate and event-free survival (EFS) rate were identical in the two arms of the study, but the overall survival (OS) was superior in the melphalan-only arm. Patients on melphalan only also experienced significantly less toxicity.

Desikan et al. performed a retrospective pairmate analysis between patients receiving melphalan (140 mg/m^2) with TBI or cyclophosphamide and patients matched for standard prognostic features and receiving melphalan (200 mg/m^2) [20]. The TBI-containing regimen failed to show any improvement in treatment response, and reported increased morbidity, increased treatment-related mortality, and inferior OS outcomes to the melphalan alone regimen. In this study, the poor outcome seen with TBI was considered to be related to delayed immune recovery.

Many other regimens that are commonly used in leukemia (busulfan–cyclophosphamide, cyclophosphamide–TBI), lymphoma (BEAM [carmustine, etoposide, cytarabine, melphalan], CBV [cyclophosphamide, carmustine, etoposide] [22,23]), and solid tumors (carboplatin–etoposide–cyclophosphamide) have been tried in MM. None of these regimens have shown superiority over melphalan alone in analyses of EBMT or American Bone Marrow Transplant registry data [24]. In general, MM patients tend to be aged >60 years, have subtle or overt renal impairment, and, not infrequently, have had prior exposure to radiation. These characteristics have precluded the widespread use of these alternative regimens.

Transplantation

Salvage therapy

In the 1980s, several investigators studied the role of high-dose chemotherapy (HDT) in relapsed and refractory MM (see **Table 1**). The dose-intensive regimen was supported by growth factors, autologous BM transplantation, and subsequently mobilized peripheral blood stem cells (PBSCs). A progressive shortening of the duration of myelosuppression, with a commensurate decline in treatment-related mortality, was observed. Dose escalation resulted in a higher response rate, which translated into better EFS and OS. Chemotherapy sensitivity at the time of HDT is an important prognostic factor for EFS and OS, although HDT is effective when applied early in

Study	Regimen	Transplant type	Prior therapy	*N*	Median age (years)	Early death (%)	CR (%)	Median EFS time (years)	Median OS time (years)
Cunningham et al. [4]	CTX 400 mg/m^2, melphalan 140 mg/m^2	ABMT	–	63	48	14	32	1.5	4
Cunningham et al. [5]	Melphalan 200 mg/m^2	ABMT	–	53	52	2	75	2.0	6.7
Anderson et al. [8]	Melphalan–TBI	ABMT (purged cells)	–/+	52	49	2	40	2.6	4.2
Bensinger et al. [6]	Busulfan–cyclophosphamide ± TBI	PBSC, ABMT	+	63	51	25	30	0.8	2.8
Bjorkstrand et al. [7]	Melphalan ± TBI	PBSC, ABMT	+	207	49	4	46	2.4	2.7
Fermand et al. [11]	TBI–CC	PBSC	–/+	63	44	11	20	3.6	6.4
Harousseau et al. [9]	Melphalan–TBI	PBSC, ABMT	–	133	52	4	37	2.0	3.8
Barlogie et al. [10]	Melphalan 200 mg/m^2 × 2	PBSC	–	231	51	2	41	3.6	5.7

Table 1. Results of high-dose chemotherapy trials in multiple myeloma. ABMT: autologous bone marrow transplantation; CC: combination chemotherapy consisting of carmustine, etoposide, melphalan, and cyclophosphamide; CR: complete remission; CTX: cyclophosphamide; EFS: event-free survival; OS: overall survival; PBSC: peripheral blood stem cells; TBI: total body irradiation; –/+: includes patients both with and without prior therapy. Adapted from [1].

the course of primary unresponsive disease (disease that does not respond to standard induction therapy).

Vesole et al. studied 135 patients with advanced refractory MM who were given high-dose chemotherapy, and reported EFS and OS times of 21 and >43 months, respectively [25]. Patients with primary unresponsive disease had superior outcomes to patients with resistant relapse (those progressing on last-salvage chemotherapy), with EFS times of 37 months versus 17 months, respectively (P = 0.0004), and OS times of ≥43 months versus 21 months, respectively (P = 0.0003) [25]. The Mayo clinic also reported a similar experience in 64 patients who had their stem cells harvested early but their transplant delayed electively until the time of progression [26].

Initial therapy

In his initial report on high-dose melphalan at 140 mg/m^2, McElwain reported three "CRs" among five previously untreated patients. This encouraging result was followed by a larger study, which included 63 previously untreated patients [4]. In all patients, a priming dose of intravenous cyclophosphamide (400 mg/m^2) was administered 7 days before melphalan. The overall response rate was 82%, with 32% of patients achieving complete remission. With longer follow-up, the investigators reported a median remission duration of 52 months for responders; and the median survival time of the entire group was 47 months [4].

By the early 1990s, the availability of growth factors and PBSC support reduced treatment-related mortality to <5%, paving the way for formal evaluation of HDT in the management of MM. Attal et al. were the first to conduct a multicenter, randomized clinical trial comparing 1 year of standard-dose chemotherapy with a short course of standard-dose induction chemotherapy followed by consolidation with HDT consisting of melphalan and TBI plus autologous BM rescue [27]. The conventional chemotherapy regimen consisted of VMCP (vincristine, melphalan, cyclophosphamide, and prednisone) alternating with

Response category	Therapy		P value
	Conventional chemotherapy	High-dose chemotherapy	
Complete remission rate	5%	22%	0.001
Complete remission + VGPR rate	14%	38%	<0.001
Median EFS time	18 months	28 months	0.01
EFS rate at 7 years	8%	16%	0.01
Median OS time	44 months	57 months	0.03
OS rate at 7 years	25%	43%	0.03

Table 2. Results from the Intergroupe Francophone du Myelome (IFM) 90 study showing the superiority of high-dose therapy with bone marrow rescue over conventional-dose chemotherapy in 200 newly diagnosed patients [27]. EFS: event-free survival; OS: overall survival; VGPR: very good partial remission.

BVAP (carmustine, vincristine, doxorubicin, and prednisone). Previously untreated patients ($N = 200$) under the age of 65 years participated in this trial. Patients randomized to transplantation had a higher CR rate (22% vs. 5%), EFS time (median 28 months vs. 18 months), and OS time (median 57 months vs. 44 months) than patients on standard-dose chemotherapy (see **Table 2** and **Figure 1**).

Similarly, the Medical Research Council (MRC)-VII trial randomized 407 patients to either standard-dose chemotherapy or HDT with transplantation. The CR rate, EFS, and OS were significantly superior in the patients receiving HDT [28]. A Spanish trial comparing standard-dose chemotherapy with HDT plus transplantation showed a superior CR rate in the HDT arm, with a trend in favor of the HDT arm for EFS and OS (see **Table 3**) [29]. Fermand et al. conducted another clinical trial in which 190 newly diagnosed MM patients aged 55–65 years were randomized to either autotransplant or standard chemotherapy [30]. This study, however, failed to show superiority of the transplant arm.

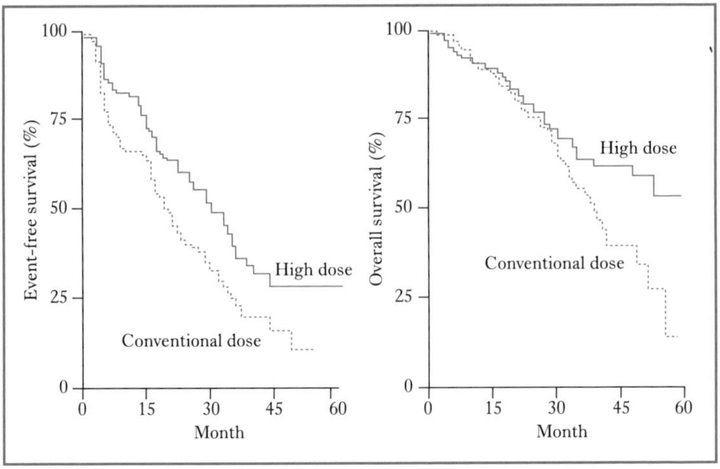

Figure 1. Intergroupe Francophone du Myelome (IFM) 90: the first randomized trial of standard VMCP (vincristine, melphalan, cyclophosphamide, and prednisone)–BVAP (carmustine, vincristine, doxorubicin, and prednisone) chemotherapy versus high-dose melphalan (140 mg/m^2) plus added total-body irradiation (8 Gy) and BM rescue. Adapted from [27].

Tandem transplants

Attempts to further improve the results of autotransplantation have included intensification with tandem transplants. Harousseau et al. were the first to report tandem autologous BM transplantation in 97 patients – 44 with advanced and 53 with newly diagnosed MM [31]. After a first administration of high-dose melphalan at 140 mg/m^2, the overall response and CR rates were 71% and 25%, respectively, with a treatment-related mortality rate of 8%. Of the 69 responders, only 35 patients had adequate autologous BM harvested to proceed with a second transplantation. Approximately half of these patients received the same dose of melphalan again, while the other half additionally received TBI. At the end of the tandem transplants, 24 patients (69%) were in CR. The OS time for the entire group of 97 patients was only 24 months, while the subset of 35 patients receiving a tandem autograft showed a modest gain in median survival time to 41 months.

Study	N	Median follow-up (months)	Median EFS time (months)		Median OS time (months)	
			CC	HDT	CC	HDT
IFM 90 [27]	200	84	18	28	44	57
MAG 91 [30]	190	56	19	24	50	55
PETHEMA[1] [29]	164	42	34	43	64	72
MRC VII [28]	407	42	20	32	42	54

Table 3. Conventional chemotherapy (CC) versus high-dose chemotherapy (HDT) in four randomized studies. EFS: event-free survival; IFM: Intergroupe Francophone du Myelome; MAG: Myelome Autogreffe Group; MRC: Medical Research Council; OS: overall survival; PETHEMA: Program for the Study and Treatment of Hematological Malignancies, Spanish Society of Hematology.
[1]In patients responding to CC and two courses of melphalan 100 mg/m^2.

However, this study was limited by:

- an inability to collect adequate autologous BM for a second autograft following the first transplant
- delayed hematopoietic recovery due to a lack of growth factors
- the use of BM for autografts, which resulted in significant delays in hematopoietic recovery, with attendant morbidity and mortality

The availability of growth factors and PBSCs for hematopoietic rescue has made autotransplants safe and feasible for the majority of MM patients involved in testing the role of tandem transplants. Barlogie et al. investigated a sequential noncross-resistant remission induction regimen followed by tandem autologous transplantations ("total therapy") in newly diagnosed patients aged <70 years [10]. Among the 231 patients who participated in this study, 84% completed one transplant and 71% completed two. There was a progressive increase in CR rate from 15% after induction to 26% after the first transplant, and 41% after two transplants. The median EFS and OS times were 43 months and 68 months, respectively. The superiority of total therapy over standard-dose chemotherapy was confirmed in a pairmate analysis comparing 116 patients treated in the tandem transplant arm with a similar number of patients treated with standard-dose chemotherapy in various Southwest Oncology Group studies [32]. Compared with standard-dose chemotherapy, tandem transplants induced a higher PR rate (86% vs. 52%; $P = 0.0001$), and extended the EFS time (49 months vs. 22 months; $P = 0.0001$), and OS time (>62 months vs. 48 month; $P = 0.01$), with a projected 5-year EFS rate of 36% versus 19% and an OS rate of 61% versus 39% [32].

The role of tandem transplantation in achieving a higher response rate and improving survival time has been investigated by the IFM group in a randomized comparison of single HDT (melphalan [140 mg/m^2] and TBI [8 Gy]) versus double HDT (melphalan [200 mg/m^2], followed by melphalan [140 mg/m^2] and TBI [8 Gy]) [33]. Between 1994 and 1997, 405 newly diagnosed patients were randomized to receive either single or double HDT after initial cytoreduction with VAD (vincristine, doxorubicin, dexamethasone). In both arms, patients underwent a second randomization at the time of receiving the TBI-containing regimen to receive either PBSCs or BM, thus dividing the patients into four groups. The results of this study, summarized in **Tables 4** and **5**, show that patients receiving tandem HDT with PBSCs have a superior outcome to those receiving single HDT. Three other randomized studies, listed in **Table 6**, are currently investigating a similar question. The Myelome Autogreffe Group (MAG) ($N = 193$), Dutch–Belgian Hematology–Oncology Cooperative Group ($N = 255$), and Bologna ($N = 178$) trials – all with a median follow-up of 27–30 months – have not yet shown a significant difference in survival for tandem transplantation. However, all of the studies require longer follow-up to draw more definitive conclusions.

	Single HDT (n = 199)	Double HDT (n = 200)
Feasibility		
HDM 140	–	88%
HDM 140 + TBI	85%	78%
Toxic death	3 patients	7 patients
Response		
HDM 140		
Response	–	77%
Complete remission	–	15%
HDM 140 + TBI		
Response	84%	82%
Complete remission	34%	35%
VGPR + complete remission	42%	49%

Table 4. Results from the Intergroupe Francophone du Myelome (IFM) 94 randomized study comparing the efficacy of single versus double high-dose chemotherapy with autologous transplantation in newly diagnosed patients with multiple myeloma [33]. HDM 140: high-dose melphalan (140 mg/m^2); TBI: total-body irradiation; VGPR: very good partial remission.

	Single HDT (n = 199)	Double HDT (n = 200)	*P* value
EFS			
Median time	31 months	37 months	0.03
6-year rate	19%	28%	
OS			
Median time	50 months	58 months	0.02
6-year rate	26%	46%	

Table 5. Survival results from the Intergroupe Francophone du Myelome (IFM) 94 study comparing the efficacy of single versus double high-dose chemotherapy (HDT) with autologous transplantation in newly diagnosed patients with myeloma [33]. EFS: event-free survival; OS: overall survival.

Study	N	Median follow-up (months)	Results
IFM 94	399	60	Better EFS and OS times with double HDT
HOVON[1]	261	33	Higher complete remission rate with double HDT (28% vs. 11%)
Bologna	178	30	No difference
MAG 95	228	40	No difference

Table 6. Preliminary results from four randomized studies assessing single versus double high-dose chemotherapy (HDT). EFS: event-free survival; HOVON: Dutch–Belgian Hematology–Oncology Cooperative Group; IFM: Intergroupe Francophone du Myelome; MAG: Myelome Autogreffe Group; OS: overall survival.
[1]2 × 70 mg/m^2 melphalan ± cyclophosphamide + total body irradiation + peripheral blood stem cell transplantation.

Timing

Treatment with curative intent is best applied during initial therapy. Therefore, transplantation should be considered as part of the initial treatment strategy rather than for recurrent disease. However, MM patients are often aged >60 years and frequently have renal impairment. Transplantation applied as part of the initial therapy prolongs remission duration and survival, but is not curative. These constraints led to the exploration of early versus delayed use of HDT in the management of MM.

In a French multicenter trial, 185 newly diagnosed patients <56 years of age received CHOP (cyclophosphamide, hydroxydaunomycin, vincristine, and prednisone) chemotherapy followed by blood progenitor cell harvesting. Subsequently, the patients were randomly assigned to receive 3–4 cycles of VAMP (vinblastine, doxorubicin, methotrexate, and prednisone) followed by HDT and autotransplantation, or conventional chemotherapy with VMCP for 1 year. In the latter group, patients were offered HDT if they had primary refractory disease, or upon relapse. Although patients who underwent early transplantation had significantly longer EFS times (39 months vs. 13 months), there was no difference in OS times [34]. However, the time without symptoms and treatment analysis reflecting quality of life showed superior results for the early HDT arm.

Hematopoietic stem cell source

Mobilized PBSCs have replaced BM stem cells (BMSCs) as the favored source of stem cells because they provide faster engraftment. The IFM 90 study has confirmed that rapid hematopoietic recovery reduces the risk of serious infections with PBSC support [27], while the EFS and OS durations were found to be similar with both types of hematopoietic support. MM patients who had received <1 year of prior therapy had faster granulocyte and platelet recovery after PBSC transplants than with BM autografts. The duration of prior chemotherapy, especially in relation to stem cell-damaging agents (eg, melphalan, carmustine, and cyclophosphamide) and radiation to BM-containing areas, significantly affects both the ability to procure adequate quantities of PBSCs and the posttransplant engraftment kinetics. Additionally, the ability to collect an adequate number of stem cells decreases as the duration of standard-dose chemotherapy increases [35]. In one study, 86% of patients with <12 months of prior therapy successfully mobilized an adequate number of stem cells ($\geq 2 \times 10^6$ $CD34^+$ cells/kg), compared with 48% of patients with >24 months of prior therapy (see **Figure 2**) [36].

Stem cell purging

Contamination of stem cells with myeloma cells has been universally shown to be detectable by polymerase chain reaction and immunofluorescence studies [37]. Various investigators have evaluated the role of tumor cell purging by positive selection of $CD34^+$ cells (leading to a 3–5 log reduction in contamination) or negative selection by the monoclonal antibody cocktail containing CD10 (common acute lymphoblastic leukemia antigen), CD20 (a pan-B cell antigen), plasma cell-associated antigen-1 or peanut agglutinin, and anti-CD19 antibodies. These purging methods resulted in there being no myeloma cells detectable by flow

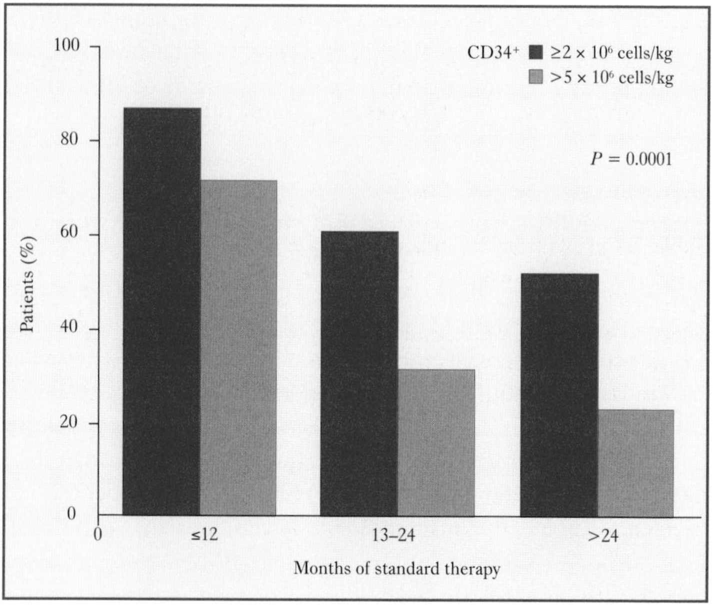

Figure 2. Hematopoietic stem cell damage with prolonged prior standard-dose therapy. This figure illustrates the proportion of patients able to mobilize $\geq 2 \times 10^6$ $CD34^+$ cells/kg and $>5 \times 10^6$ $CD34^+$ cells/kg after ≤12, 13–24, and >24 months of prior therapy ($N = 542$).

cytometry [8,38]. Despite the success at obtaining a tumor-free graft via purging, the follow-up results from various pilot studies have not revealed any significant advantage in response or survival time, and there is a posttransplantation delay in engraftment [8,39]. A large, multicenter, randomized study comparing CD34-selected cells versus unselected PBSCs in 131 patients failed to show any significant prolongation of EFS or OS time with selection (see **Table 7**) [38]. However, timely neutrophil and platelet recovery was observed in patients receiving CD34-selected PBSCs. In a study selecting very early hematopoietic stem cells ($CD34^+$, $Thy1^+$, Lin^-) devoid of any clonal B cell contamination, relapses were frequent and patients had delayed hematopoietic engraftment and prolonged suppressed immune status with associated infectious complications [39].

	Selected cells	Unselected cells	*P* value
Median OS time	50 months	Not reached	0.78
Median DFS time	100 weeks	104 weeks	0.82
Relapse rate	67%	66%	–
Mortality rate	36%	35%	–

Table 7. Results from an update of a Phase III study (n = 190) showing a lack of improvement in survival times with CD34 selection. The reduction in tumor burden was 1.6–6.0 log (median 3.1) following CD34 selection and there were no detected tumor cells in 54% of patients. No significant differences were observed in time to count recovery, number of transfusions, transplant-related mortality, and days in hospital [38]. DFS: Disease-free survival; OS: overall survival.

As CR is observed in only 30%–50% of patients, greater emphasis needs to be placed on achieving tumor cytoreduction.

Patient selection

Older patients

The role of HDT has been evaluated in patients >65 years old, as incidence of MM increases with advancing age (median age 64 years). No significant differences in clinical characteristics have been observed between younger and older patients, and age has not been reported to affect stem cell mobilization or engraftment [40]. Badros et al. evaluated the feasibility and efficacy of HDT with PBSC transplant in patients ≥70 years old [41]. In 70 patients (median age 72 years; range 70–83 years) treated with melphalan (200 mg/m^2 or 140 mg/m^2), 27% CR was achieved after tandem transplants. Median CR duration was 1.5 years, and 3-year EFS and OS rates were projected at 20% and 31%, respectively. However, treatment-related mortality was higher (16%) in the initial 25 patients receiving melphalan at 200 mg/m^2. Although this study confirms the feasibility of HDT in older patients with MM, it also indicates a higher risk in this patient population, and the need for strict patient selection based on clinical status.

Patients with renal failure

Over one-third of MM patients have reversible renal dysfunction in the initial stages of the disease. With effective therapy, there is a likelihood of recovery in almost half of patients. High-dose melphalan, with its pharmacokinetics independent of renal function, has been evaluated in MM patients with renal dysfunction. In a study by Badros et al., 81 patients with MM and renal failure (creatinine >2 mg/dL) at the time of autologous SCT (38 patients were on dialysis) were treated with high-dose melphalan and PBSC transplantation [42]. In this setting, renal failure had no impact on the quality of stem cell collection and/or engraftment. Treatment-related mortality rates were 6% and 13% after the first and second autologous SCTs, respectively. Complete remission was achieved in 31 patients (38%) after tandem SCT. Two patients discontinued dialysis after autologous PBSC transplantation. The probabilities of EFS and OS to 3 years were 48% and 55%, respectively. Although melphalan at 200 mg/m^2 caused excessive toxicity, melphalan at 140 mg/m^2 was better tolerated.

A short time to CR correlates with a higher chance of recovery of renal function. The role of transplantation in the setting of renal failure remains investigational, and dose reduction and close monitoring are needed to ensure the safety of the procedure.

Factors predicting outcome

Various prognostic indicators have been investigated to find a good predictor of outcome following HDT and autologous SCT. These factors include:

- β_2-microglobulin
- the plasma cell labeling index
- cytogenetic abnormalities (particularly deletion or translocations affecting chromosome 13)

- lactate dehydrogenase
- C-reactive protein

Barlogie et al. evaluated the role of tandem transplantation in 231 newly diagnosed patients with MM and reported the absence or deletion of the q arm of chromosome 13 and a high serum β_2-microglobulin level (>2.5 mg/L) to be the two most important factors predicting shorter EFS and OS [10]. Desikan et al. evaluated more than 1,000 patients undergoing HDT and identified C-reactive protein concentration of ≤4 mg/L, a serum β_2-microglobulin concentration of ≤2.5 mg/L, and <12 months of therapy prior to HDT as favorable prognostic indicators [43].

A review of serial cytogenetic studies in all patients revealed that chromosome 13 deletion was the only prognostic cytogenetic variable [43]. This variable was independent of, and ranked higher than, the standard prognostic factors for both EFS and OS. The significance of chromosome 13 abnormalities has been confirmed using interphase fluorescence *in situ* hybridization (FISH) with a retinoblastoma gene-1 (*rb-1*)-specific probe (13q14) in 97 consecutive patients with MM [44]. In a retrospective analysis by the IFM group of 110 patients undergoing HDT, detection of chromosome 13 abnormalities by FISH was strongly predictive of adverse outcome, along with a high β_2-microglobulin level (>2.5 mg/L) and immunoglobulin A isotype [45].

Maintenance therapy

There is no clear plateau in the survival curve, despite increased remission rates with HDT. In an effort to sustain remission, various maintenance therapies have been evaluated in MM. IFN-α has been the most widely investigated treatment, although randomized studies have only demonstrated modest improvements in EFS and OS times (5–12 months) in patients achieving remission with standard-dose therapy. Its role following HDT has not been confirmed [46]. Similarly, the role of maintenance prednisone given on alternate days to prolong survival has been confirmed by a randomized study following standard-dose therapy; however, its role in the setting of HDT needs confirmation [47]. Additional new approaches for maintenance are under investigation, including the role of thalidomide with and without added dexamethasone, bisphosphonates, and immune manipulations such as idiotype vaccination and protein-pulsed dendritic cell-based vaccination strategies.

Allogeneic transplantation

The first attempts at transplantation in MM were between identical twins. Bensinger et al. reported the largest single-center experience on syngeneic transplants [48]. Of the 11 patients receiving transplants, five achieved CR and three achieved PR. At the time of the report, one patient from each remission group was alive, 9 years and 15 years after transplantation, respectively.

Gahrton et al. reviewed the EBMT Registry data of 25 patients who had undergone twin transplants, and compared their outcome by case-matched analysis to 125 patients each undergoing autotransplantation or allogeneic transplantation [49]. The complete remission rate was not significantly different between the three grafts (twin: 68%; autologous: 48%; allogeneic: 58%). However, the median survival time was significantly superior for syngeneic transplantation compared with autologous (72 months vs. 25 months; $P = 0.009$) or allogeneic (72 months vs. 16 months; $P = 0.008$) transplantation.

Donor availability, frequent renal impairment, and a restriction to patients under 60 years of age has limited the use of matched sibling transplantation in MM. Tumor-free graft and possible graft-versus-myeloma (GVM) effect should result in a favorable outcome after allogeneic transplantation. Supportive evidence includes higher molecular CR and a lower relapse rate following allogeneic rather than autologous transplants.

A retrospective case-matched analysis of EBMT registry data acquired before 1995 comparing 189 patients receiving allografts with an equal number of patients receiving autotransplants during the same period showed a better survival outcome for patients who had autotransplants [50]. The median survival time after allogeneic transplants was 18 months, compared with 34 months after autotransplants. The poor outcome was related to transplant-related mortality: 41% with allotransplants and 13% with autotransplants. Patients who survived the first year following allotransplants had a tendency for better progression-free survival and OS times.

There has been a reduction in transplant-related mortality over time. An update of the EBMT registry results by Gahrton et al. indicates a reduction in transplant-related mortality after 1994, mainly due to better selection of patients, ie, those with less prior chemotherapy. Even so, the transplant-related mortality rate was 30% at 2 years [51]. The use of PBSCs has resulted in speedier engraftment, but has not improved outcomes. Long-term follow-up also indicates no plateau in the survival curve after allotransplantation.

A single-center result from the Dana-Farber Cancer Institute reported a very low transplant-related mortality of 10% due to selective depletion of $CD6^+$ T cells as the only form of graft-versus-host disease (GvHD) prophylaxis [52]. However, the median progression-free survival time was 12 months, and the median OS time was 22 months. These results were inferior to those found by the investigators in their previous experience of autologous transplantation. Case-matched comparative studies from other single institutions have also failed to show a survival advantage for allotransplants.

Investigators at the University of Arkansas compared their results from 42 patients undergoing allotransplants after failing a single autotransplant with 42 pair-matched controls who had salvage autotransplantation under identical conditions. The CR rate

(41% vs. 33%) and 3-year probability of EFS (25% vs. 20%) were comparable between the two transplant types, but the 3-year probability of survival favored autotransplantation (54% vs. 29%; $P = 0.013$) [53].

Donor lymphocyte infusions

A GVM effect has been demonstrated by the induction of CR with donor lymphocyte infusion (DLI) following relapse after allogeneic transplantation. Lokhorst et al. described 27 patients who received 52 DLIs at a median of 30 months after their previous allotransplant [54]. Six patients achieved CR and eight achieved PR. Five patients were disease-free more than 30 months after DLI. GvHD was the major side effect, and was encountered in acute form in 55% and chronic form in 26% of patients. Five patients experienced BM aplasia, and two of them died from it.

Salama et al. reported DLI experiences in 25 MM patients from 15 centers in the US [55]. The DLIs were performed in patients with persistent or recurrent disease following an allogeneic transplantation. A total of 10 patients responded, four with CR and six with PR. Acute GvHD was seen in 13 of the 25 patients, while 11 of the 21 evaluable patients developed chronic GvHD.

Several strategies have been explored to reduce GvHD after DLI [56,57]:

- lowering the number of T cell infusions
- selective depletion of $CD8^+$ T cells
- herpes simplex virus (HSV) thymidine kinase-gene transduction of DLI

Infusion of $<1 \times 10^7$ T cells is not associated with GvHD. However, there is also no GVM effect observed following infusion of $<1 \times 10^8$ T cells. The removal of $CD8^+$ cells does not eliminate GvHD. Experimental evidence suggests that a population of

T cells that induces a GVM effect exists and is distinct from the T cells that induce GvHD, though it has not been possible to assess this effectively in a clinical setting. Immunizing donors with idiotype vaccine may allow selective transfer of T cells specific for GVM without increasing the incidence of GvHD.

Nonmyeloablative transplants

For a long time, BM ablation coupled with immunosuppression was considered to be a prerequisite for allogeneic progenitor cell engraftment. However, studies in a canine model demonstrated that the dose of TBI could be reduced to nonmyeloablative levels with successful engraftment when used in conjunction with a combination of cyclosporin and mycophenolate mofetil [58]. Thus, immunosuppression to avoid GvHD was also able to prevent graft rejection (host-versus-graft reaction). This reduced day 100 transplant-related mortality and allowed allogeneic-matched sibling transplantation in patients over the age of 50 years and/or patients who were otherwise considered high risk for the standard allogeneic preparative regimen.

Investigators from the University of Arkansas reported 16 high-risk patients with MM who received allogeneic transplants from human leukocyte antigen-matched (n = 14) or mismatched (n = 2) donors following nonmyeloablative conditioning with melphalan (100 mg/m^2). Transplant-related mortality in the first 120 days was low (6%). Acute GvHD developed in 10 patients (63%) – with one resultant fatality – and chronic GvHD was seen in seven patients (44%) living beyond 4 months, of whom four (25%) had extensive GvHD and one died. In this preliminary report with a short follow-up period (2–18 months), seven patients were alive, and five were in CR [59].

Maloney et al. reported the feasibility of autotransplantation for tumor cytoreduction followed by nonmyeloablative matched sibling transplantation in 32 patients [60]. The mortality rate for the first 100 days was low (6%), and the treatment could essentially be performed in an outpatient setting. The response rate was 84% (53% CR) and the 1-year survival rate was >80%. Acute or chronic GvHD was encountered in 55% of patients.

Giralt et al. reported the use of reduced intensity conditioning with fludarabine and melphalan followed by allogeneic transplantation in patients with MM. Although all patients engrafted successfully, the 100-day mortality rate was 20% and the 1-year mortality rate was 40%, with six patients alive after a median follow-up period of 15 months [61].

Nonmyeloablative transplants are still associated with significant morbidity due to acute and chronic GvHD and a mortality rate of 20% at 1 year [62]. While the early clinical results are encouraging, long-term follow-up results are required before nonmyeloablative transplantation can be universally recommended for all patients with a matched sibling donor.

Conclusions

HDT with PBSC support can be applied safely in MM and achieves significantly higher CR rates as well as statistically superior EFS and OS times than standard-dose combination chemotherapy. However, neither tumor-cell purging, intensification of conditioning with additional chemotherapeutic agents, nor TBI have been shown to improve outcomes. Advanced age (>65 years) and renal failure are not absolute contraindications for HDT with PBSC support. The role of tandem transplantation with high-dose melphalan is being evaluated by various groups in a randomized study. Although only one study has demonstrated evidence of superior outcomes, longer follow-up is required for a more definite conclusion. Along with HDT, future research will include combining the best current remission-induction regimens with maintenance treatments (eg, thalidomide, idiotype or dendritic cell-based vaccination) that will sustain CR. Development of nonmyeloablative allogeneic transplantation for safer application of GVM effect provides an alternative strategy, in select patients, to achieve long-term disease-free survival.

References

1. Munshi NC, Tricot T, Barlogie BB. Plasma cell neoplasms. In: DeVita VT, Rosenberg SA, Hellman S, editors. *Cancer: Principles and Practice of Oncology* (6th edition). New York, NY: Lippincott, Williams & Wilkins, 2000:2465–98.
2. McElwain TJ, Powles RL. High-dose intravenous melphalan for plasma-cell leukemia and myeloma. *Lancet* 1983;2:822–4.
3. Frei E 3rd, Antman K, Teicher B et al. Bone marrow autotransplantation for solid tumors – prospects. *J Clin Oncol* 1989;7:515–26.
4. Cunningham D, Paz-Ares L, Milan S et al. High-dose melphalan and autologous bone marrow transplantation as consolidation in previously untreated myeloma. *J Clin Oncol* 1994;12:759–63.
5. Cunningham D, Paz-Ares L, Gore ME et al. High-dose melphalan for multiple myeloma: long-term follow-up data. *J Clin Oncol* 1994;12:764–8.
6. Bensinger WI, Rowley SD, Demirer T et al. High-dose therapy followed by autologous hematopoietic stem-cell infusion for patients with multiple myeloma. *J Clin Oncol* 1996;14:1447–56.
7. Bjorkstrand B, Ljungman P, Bird JM et al. Autologous stem cell transplantation in multiple myeloma: results of the European Group for Bone Marrow Transplantation. *Stem Cells* 1995;13(Suppl. 2):140–6.
8. Anderson KC, Anderson J, Soiffer R et al. Monoclonal antibody-purged bone marrow transplantation therapy for multiple myeloma. *Blood* 1993;82:2568–76.
9. Harousseau JL, Attal M, Divine M et al. Autologous stem cell transplantation after first remission induction treatment in multiple myeloma. A report of the French Registry on Autologous Transplantation in Multiple Myeloma. *Stem Cells* 1995;13(Suppl. 2):132–9.
10. Barlogie B, Jagannath S, Desikan KR et al. Total therapy with tandem transplants for newly diagnosed multiple myeloma. *Blood* 1999;93:55–65.
11. Fermand JP, Ravaud P, Chevret S et al. High-dose therapy and autologous blood stem cell transplantation in multiple myeloma: preliminary results of a randomized trial involving 167 patients. *Stem Cells* 1995;13(Suppl. 2):156–9.
12. Barlogie B, Alexanian R, Dicke KA et al. High-dose chemoradiotherapy and autologous bone marrow transplantation for resistant multiple myeloma. *Blood* 1987;70:869–72.
13. Tricot G, Alberts DS, Johnson C et al. Safety of autotransplants with high-dose melphalan in renal failure: a pharmacokinetic and toxicity study. *Clin Cancer Res* 1996;2:947–52.
14. Jagannath S, Vesole DH, Tricot G et al. Hemopoietic stem cell transplants for multiple myeloma. *Oncology (Huntingt)* 1994;8:89–103; discussion 103–6.
15. Jagannath S, Barlogie B. Autologous bone marrow transplantation for multiple myeloma. *Hematol Oncol Clin North Am* 1992;6:437–49.
16. Moreau P, Milpied N, Mahe B et al. Melphalan 220 mg/m^2 followed by peripheral blood stem cell transplantation in 27 patients with advanced multiple myeloma. *Bone Marrow Transplant* 1999;23:1003–6.
17. Fermand JP, Levy Y, Gerota J et al. Treatment of aggressive multiple myeloma by high-dose chemotherapy and total body irradiation followed by blood stem cells autologous graft. *Blood* 1989;73:20–3.
18. Anderson KC, Barut BA, Ritz J et al. Monoclonal antibody-purged autologous bone marrow transplantation therapy for multiple myeloma. *Blood* 1991;77:712–20.
19. Abraham R, Chen C, Tsang R et al. Intensification of the stem cell transplant induction regimen results in increased treatment-related mortality without improved outcome in multiple myeloma. *Bone Marrow Transplant* 1999;24:1291–7.

20. Desikan KR, Tricot G, Dhodapkar M et al. Melphalan plus total body irradiation (MEL-TBI) or cyclophosphamide (MEL-CY) as a conditioning regimen with second autotransplant in responding patients with myeloma is inferior compared to historical controls receiving tandem transplants with melphalan alone. *Bone Marrow Transplant* 2000;25:483–7.
21. Moreau P, Facon T, Attal M. Comparison of 200 mg/m^2 melphalan and 8 Gy total body irradiation plus 140 mg/m^2 melphalan as conditioning regimens for peripheral blood stem cell transplantation in patients with newly diagnosed multiple myeloma: final analysis of the Intergroupe Francophone du Myelome 9502 randomized trial. *Blood* 2002;99:731–5.
22. Ventura GJ, Barlogie B, Hester JP et al. High dose cyclophosphamide, BCNU and VP-16 with autologous blood stem cell support for refractory multiple myeloma. *Bone Marrow Transplant* 1990;5:265–8.
23. Adkins DR, Salzman D, Boldt D et al. Phase I trial of dacarbazine with cyclophosphamide, carmustine, etoposide, and autologous stem-cell transplantation in patients with lymphoma and multiple myeloma. *J Clin Oncol* 1994;12:1890–901.
24. Bjorkstrand B. European Group for Blood and Marrow Transplantation Registry studies in multiple myeloma. *Semin Hematol* 2001;38:219–25.
25. Vesole DH, Barlogie B, Jagannath S et al. High-dose therapy for refractory multiple myeloma: improved prognosis with better supportive care and double transplants. *Blood* 1994;84:950–6.
26. Gertz MA, Lacy MQ, Inwards DJ et al. Early harvest and late transplantation as an effective therapeutic strategy in multiple myeloma. *Bone Marrow Transplant* 1999;23:221–6.
27. Attal M, Harousseau JL, Stoppa AM et al. A prospective, randomized trial of autologous bone marrow transplantation and chemotherapy in multiple myeloma. Intergroupe Francais du Myelome. *N Engl J Med* 1996;335:91–7.
28. Child JA, Morgan GJ, Davies FE et al. High-dose chemotherapy with hematopoietic stem-cell rescue for multiple myeloma. *N Eng J Med* 2003;348:1875–83.
29. Bladé J, Sureda A, Ribera JM et al. High-dose therapy autotransplantation/intensification vs continued conventional chemotherapy in multiple myeloma in patients responding to initial treatment chemotherapy: results of a prospective randomized trial from the Spanish Cooperative Group (PETHEMA). *Blood* 2001;98:815a.
30. Fermand JP, Ravaud P, Katsahian S et al. High dose therapy and autologous blood stem cell transplantation versus conventional treatment in multiple myeloma: results of a randomized trial in 190 patients 55 to 65 years of age. *Blood* 1999;94 (Suppl. 1):396a.
31. Harousseau JL, Milipied N, Laporte JP et al. Double-intensive therapy in high-risk multiple myeloma. *Blood* 1992;79:2827–33.
32. Barlogie B, Jagannath S, Vesole DH et al. Superiority of tandem autologous transplantation over standard therapy for previously untreated multiple myeloma. *Blood* 1997;89:789–93.
33. Attal M, Harousseau JL, Facon T et al. Double autologous transplantation improves survival of multiple myeloma patients: final analysis of a prospective randomized study of the "Intergroupe Francophone du Myelome" (IFM 94). *Blood* 2002;100:7a.
34. Fermand J-P, Ravaud P, Chevret S et al. High-dose therapy and autologous peripheral blood stem cell transplantation in multiple myeloma: up-front or rescue treatment? Results of a multicenter sequential randomized clinical trial. *Blood* 1998;92:3131–6.
35. Desikan KR, Barlogie B, Jagannath S et al. Comparable engraftment kinetics following peripheral-blood stem-cell infusion mobilized with granulocyte colony-stimulating factor with or without cyclophosphamide in multiple myeloma. *J Clin Oncol* 1998;16:1547–53.

36. Desikan KR, Jagannath S, Siegel D et al. Collection of more hematopoietic progenitor cells with large volume leukapheresis in patients with multiple myeloma. *Leuk Lymphoma* 1998;28:501–8.
37. Gazitt Y, Tian E, Barlogie B et al. Differential mobilization of myeloma cells and normal hematopoietic stem cells in multiple myeloma after treatment with cyclophosphamide and granulocyte-macrophage colony-stimulating factor. *Blood* 1996;87:805–11.
38. Stewart AK, Vescio R, Schiller G et al. Purging of autologous peripheral-blood stem cells using CD34 selection does not improve overall or progression-free survival following high dose chemotherapy: results of a multicenter randomized controlled trial. *J Clin Oncol* 2001;19:3771–9.
39. Tricot G, Gazitt Y, Leemhuis T et al. Collection, tumor contamination, and engraftment kinetics of highly purified hematopoietic progenitor cells to support high dose therapy in multiple myeloma. *Blood* 1998;91:4489–95.
40. Siegel DS, Desikan KR, Mehta J et al. Age is not a prognostic variable with autotransplants for multiple myeloma. *Blood* 1999;93:51–4.
41. Badros A, Barlogie B, Siegel E et al. Autologous stem cell transplantation in elderly multiple myeloma patients over the age of 70 years. *Br J Haematol* 2001;114:600–7.
42. Badros A, Barlogie B, Siegel E et al. Results of autologous stem cell transplant in multiple myeloma patients with renal failure. *Br J Haematol* 2001;114:822–9.
43. Desikan R, Barlogie B, Sawyer J et al. Results of high-dose therapy for 1000 patients with multiple myeloma: durable complete remissions and superior survival in the absence of chromosome 13 abnormalities. *Blood* 2000;95:4008–10.
44. Zojer N, Konigsberg R, Ackermann J et al. Deletion of 13q14 remains an independent adverse prognostic variable in multiple myeloma despite its frequent detection by interphase fluorescence in situ hybridization. *Blood* 2000;95:1925–30.
45. Facon T, Avet-Loiseau H, Guillerm G et al. Chromosome 13 abnormalities identified by FISH analysis and serum β_2-microglobulin produce a powerful myeloma staging system for patients receiving high-dose therapy. *Blood* 2001;97:1566–71.
46. Browman GP, Bergsagel DP, Sicheri D et al. Randomized trial of interferon maintenance in multiple myeloma: a study of the National Cancer Institute of Canada Clinical Trials Group. *J Clin Oncol* 1995;13:2354–60.
47. Berenson JR, Crowley JJ, Grogan TM et al. Maintenance therapy with alternate-day prednisone improves survival in multiple myeloma patients. *Blood* 2002;99:3163–8.
48. Bensinger WI, Demirer T, Buckner CD et al. Syngeneic marrow transplantation in patients with multiple myeloma. *Bone Marrow Transplant* 1996;18:527–31.
49. Gahrton G, Svensson H, Bjorkstrand B et al. Syngeneic transplantation in multiple myeloma – a case matched comparison with autologous and allogeneic transplantation. European Group for Blood and Marrow Transplant. *Bone Marrow Transplant* 1999;24:741–5.
50. Bjorkstrand B, Ljungman P, Svensson H et al. Allogeneic bone marrow transplantation versus autologous stem cell transplantation in multiple myeloma: a retrospective case-matched study from the European Group for Blood and Marrow Transplantation. *Blood* 1996;88:4711–8.
51. Gahrton G, Svensson H, Cavo M et al. Progress in allogeneic bone marrow and peripheral blood stem cell transplantation for multiple myeloma: a comparison between transplants performed 1983–93 and 1994–8 at European Group for Blood and Marrow Transplantation centres. *Br J Haematol* 2001;113:209–16.
52. Alyea EP, Anderson KC. Allotransplantation for multiple myeloma. *Cancer J* 2001;7:166–74.
53. Mehta J, Tricot G, Jagannath S et al. Salvage autologous or allogeneic transplantation for multiple myeloma refractory to or relapsing after a first-line autograft? *Bone Marrow Transplant* 1998;21:887–92.

54. Lokhorst HM, Schattenberg A, Cornelissen JJ et al. Donor lymphocyte infusions for relapsed multiple myeloma after allogeneic stem-cell transplantation: predictive factors for response and long-term outcome. *J Clin Oncol* 2000;18:3031–7.
55. Salama M, Nevill T, Marcellus D et al. Donor leukocyte infusions for multiple myeloma. *Bone Marrow Transplant* 2000;26:1179–84.
56. Soiffer RJ, Alyea EP, Hochberg E et al. Randomized trial of CD8$^+$ T-cell depletion in the prevention of graft-versus-host disease associated with donor lymphocyte infusion. *Biol Blood Marrow Transplant* 2002;8:625–32.
57. Munshi NC, Govindarajan R, Drake R et al. Thymidine kinase (TK) gene-transduced human lymphocytes can be highly purified, remain fully functional, and are killed efficiently with ganciclovir. *Blood* 1997;89:1334–40.
58. Storb R, Yu C, Zaucha JM et al. Stable mixed hematopoietic chimerism in dogs given donor antigen, CTLA4Ig, and 100 cGy total body irradiation before and pharmacologic immunosuppression after marrow transplant. *Blood* 1999;94:2523–9.
59. Badros A, Barlogie B, Morris C et al. High response rate in refractory and poor-risk multiple myeloma after allotransplantation using a nonmyeloablative conditioning regimen and donor lymphocyte infusions. *Blood* 2001;97:2574–9.
60. Maloney DG, Sahebi F, Stockerl-Goldstein KE et al. Combining an allogeneic graft-vs-myeloma effect with high-dose autologous stem cell rescue in the treatment of multiple myeloma. *Blood* 2001;98:434a.
61. Giralt S, Aleman A, Anagnostopoulos A et al. Fludarabine/melphalan conditioning for allogeneic transplantation in patients with multiple myeloma. *Bone Marrow Transplant* 2002;30:367–73.
62. Kroger N, Schwerdtfeger R, Kiehl M et al. Autologous stem cell transplantation followed by a dose-reduced allograft induces high complete remission rate in multiple myeloma. *Blood* 2002;100:755–60.

6

Bone disease

Jamie D Cavenagh & Peter I Croucher

Introduction

Bone disease is a major cause of morbidity and mortality in MM, and results in many of the debilitating features of the tumor. Osteolytic bone lesions cause bone pain, hypercalcemia, pathologic fractures, and reduced function. Osteopenia is a frequent finding, and can also result in pain and bone fractures. Vertebral collapse, along with the associated effects of a tumor mass, results in back pain, kyphosis, and height loss, as well as root and cord compressive events. Consequent neurologic deficits, including paraparesis, are among the most disabling complications of MM bone disease.

Unfortunately, these are all common presenting features in patients with MM. In some series, more than 50% of patients have presented with vertebral fractures, and up to 30% with nonvertebral fractures [1]. Generalized osteopenia is present in 60% of patients, of which 5% will have no associated lytic lesions [2].

It is anticipated that improved understanding of the pathogenesis of bone disease will result in better treatments to prevent these potentially devastating complications.

The normal process of bone remodeling

In the adult skeleton, bone is constantly being turned over in a process known as bone remodeling. This begins with the activation of a previously quiescent bone surface and recruitment of osteoclast precursors. The osteoclast precursor cells fuse to form multinucleated osteoclasts, which are responsible for resorbing bone. Having resorbed a quantum of bone, the osteoclasts are replaced by osteoblasts, which synthesize new bone matrix. This matrix is subsequently mineralized to replace the resorbed bone, and the bone surface returns to a state of quiescence.

The processes of resorption and formation are coupled in both time and space, with resorption always preceding formation. Under normal circumstances, the amount of bone resorbed is equal to that formed. However, with increasing age, this balance changes such that resorption exceeds formation. Therefore, in disorders characterized by an increased rate of bone loss, bone can be lost in a number of ways. These include:

- increasing the amount of bone resorbed
- reducing the amount of bone formed
- increasing the frequency with which remodeling units are activated, thereby further enhancing the extent of resorption in situations where resorption outweighs formation

Bone loss in multiple myeloma

Mechanisms

The cellular and molecular mechanisms responsible for bone disease in patients with MM are unclear. However, histomorphometric studies of bone biopsies taken from MM patients have provided valuable information about some of the cellular mechanisms that may contribute to this bone loss. These studies have demonstrated that, in MM, the proportion of bone surface undergoing resorption and the numbers of osteoclasts present may be increased [3–5]. One study demonstrated that the amount of bone resorbed within individual resorption sites may also be increased, which is consistent with an increase in the number and/or activity of osteoclasts at these sites [6].

Increased resorption has also been observed in patients with a low level of tumor infiltration of the bone marrow (BM) [5], or those defined as having early MM [4]. This raises the possibility that increased bone resorption is an early event in the disease process. Indeed, Bataille et al. have shown that a small proportion of patients with monoclonal gammopathy of undetermined significance have increased bone resorption, and it is these subjects who are most likely to develop overt MM compared with patients who have normal histologic indices of resorption [7]. Histomorphometric studies have demonstrated that bone formation may also be increased in the early stages of myeloma [4]. This is likely to reflect the tight coupling of resorption to formation. However, as the disease progresses, bone formation is decreased, leading to an increased negative remodeling balance, uncoupling of resorption and formation, and the rapid bone loss that is seen in osteolytic bone disease [4,6].

Regulation

The increased bone resorption seen in MM is associated with tumor cell infiltration, and may be correlated with tumor burden [5,8]. Histologic studies have shown that myeloma cells are closely associated with osteoclasts and bone surfaces actively undergoing resorption (see **Figure 1**). This suggests that the myeloma cells stimulate the resorption process directly, either by producing soluble factors that promote bone resorption, by interacting directly in a cell contact-dependent manner to stimulate osteoclastic bone resorption, or by influencing expression of resorption-modifying agents in the local BM microenvironment.

In early studies, Mundy et al. reported the production of an osteoclast-activating activity from human myeloma cell lines and primary cells isolated from patients with MM [9,10]. The identity of the cytokines and/or local growth factors that contribute to this

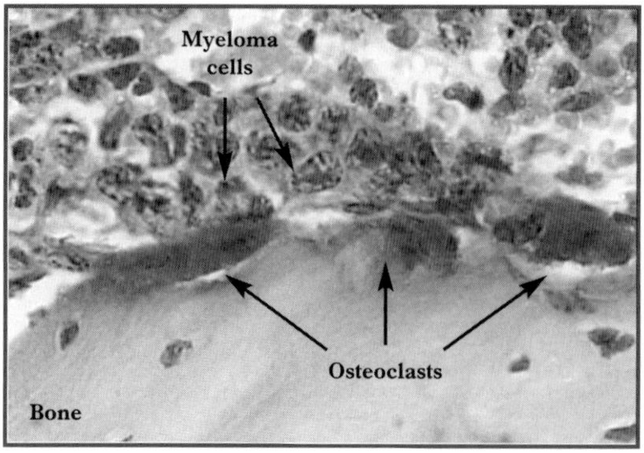

Figure 1. Histologic section showing the relationship between myeloma cells and osteoclasts. Myeloma cells can be found in close proximity to osteoclasts lining bone surfaces. Osteoclasts can be seen resorbing bone.

activity remain unclear, because different studies have implicated a range of different factors.

The reasons for the discrepancies in the different factors implicated between studies are unknown, but are likely to reflect methodological differences. These could include limitations associated with studying myeloma cell lines as opposed to primary cells, and examining whole marrow samples or preparations enriched in plasma cells to 90%–95% purity such that contaminating cells are also present. Furthermore, *in vitro* studies remove myeloma cells from the influences of the BM microenvironment, and such influences may be critical for the maintenance of an appropriate myeloma cell phenotype.

Although important differences exist between studies, a number of factors have been reported to be produced by myeloma cells, and are thus implicated in mediating the increase in bone resorption. These include a number of cytokines and growth factors, such as interleukin (IL)-1β, IL-6, lymphotoxin (LT), tumor necrosis factor (TNF)-α, macrophage inflammatory protein (MIP)-1α, and the ligand for the receptor activator of nuclear factor-κB (RANKL).

Interleukin-1β, lymphotoxin, and tumor necrosis factor-α

IL-1β is a potent bone-resorbing cytokine that is produced by BM cells isolated from MM patients [11]. It has been suggested that myeloma cells, purified from the BM of patients with MM, are responsible for the synthesis of this cytokine [12–14]. The supernatants from these enriched populations of myeloma cells have been reported to promote bone resorption in organ culture [12–14]. *In situ* hybridization studies have also shown that IL-1β mRNA is expressed by single isolated myeloma cells [15,16]. However, immunofluorescence analyses have been unable to demonstrate expression of the IL-1β protein in the same cells [16]. Furthermore, highly purified myeloma cells (>98%) are also unable to produce IL-1β [17].

Human myeloma cell lines have also been reported to produce LT, another important bone-resorbing agent [12,18,19]. However, the majority of studies have failed to demonstrate LT activity in primary myeloma cells [12,13]. Furthermore, the bone-resorbing activity that is present in cultures of these cells is not inhibited by antibodies to LT [12].

TNF-α, which is also able to stimulate bone resorption, is produced in cultures of BM cells isolated from patients with MM [11]. Furthermore, purified myeloma cells express TNF-α mRNA [18,12], and single-cell studies have detected the protein in MM cells [16].

Although IL-1β, LT, and TNF-α may be expressed by myeloma cells or produced by cells in the local BM microenvironment, there are few functional data to support a causal role in promoting osteoclast formation and bone resorption *in vivo*.

Interleukin-6

IL-6 has been established as a growth and survival factor for myeloma cells [20,21]. Studies have shown that myeloma cells may synthesize IL-6 in an autocrine manner [20,22–25] or promote its production in a paracrine manner in cells of the BM microenvironment [26,27]. IL-6 has also been shown to promote osteoclast formation in culture systems *in vitro* [28] and, at high concentrations, may promote osteoclast activity directly [29]. However, its role in promoting the development of MM bone disease remains to be established.

Macrophage inflammatory protein-1α

MIP-1α is a member of the chemokine family. It has been shown to induce the formation of osteoclasts in BM cultures, and to be chemotactic for osteoclasts. Choi et al. reported that MIP-1α is produced by myeloma cells, and that marrow plasma concentrations of MIP-1α are elevated in patients with active disease when compared with patients with early MM or those in remission [30].

Antibodies to MIP-1α inhibit the osteoclast-forming activity present in the BM plasma of patients with MM [30]. Furthermore, injection of ARH-77 cells transfected with an antisense construct to MIP-1α into severe combined immunodeficient (SCID) mice reduces osteoclast formation and inhibits the development of osteolytic lesions when compared with animals injected with control cells [31]. Interestingly, inhibition of MIP-1α was associated with a significant decrease in serum immunoglobulin (Ig)G paraprotein level, and appeared to promote an increase in mouse survival time. More recently, antibodies to MIP-1α have been shown to prevent the development of myeloma and reduce tumor burden in the 5TGM1 model of myeloma bone disease, confirming the importance of this molecule [32].

Receptor activator of NF-κB ligand

RANKL is expressed by BM stromal cells (BMSCs) and osteoblasts in the local BM microenvironment, where it can bind to its receptor RANK on the surface of osteoclast precursors [33]. The binding of RANKL to RANK plays an important role in promoting osteoclast differentiation and bone resorption [34]. A soluble decoy receptor known as osteoprotegerin (OPG), which is secreted by BM stromal cells and osteoblasts, has also

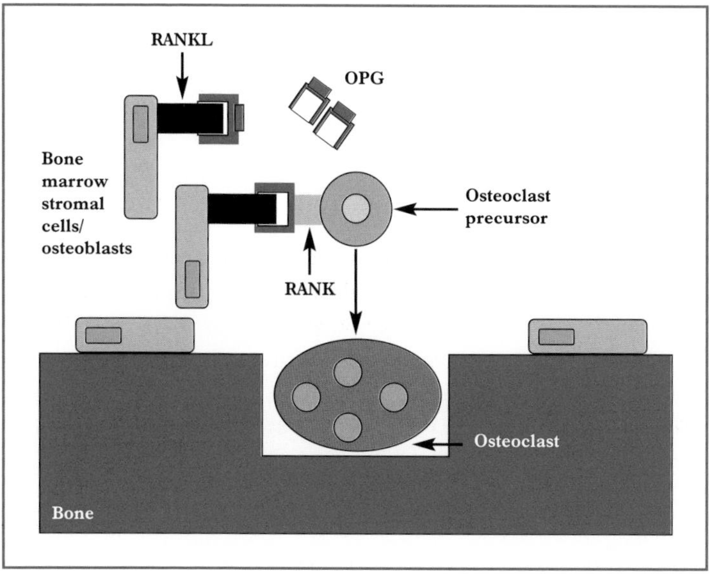

Figure 2. Diagrammatic representation of the receptor activator of nuclear factor-κB ligand (RANKL)/osteoprotegerin (OPG) system. RANKL is expressed by bone marrow stromal cells and osteoblasts. It binds to its receptor RANK on the surface of osteoclast precursors, inducing their differentiation into functional osteoclasts. OPG, a soluble decoy receptor, is also present. OPG can bind to RANKL, preventing its interaction with RANK, and thus inhibiting osteoclast formation.

been identified [35]. OPG can bind to RANKL, inhibiting its ability to bind to RANK, and preventing osteoclast formation and bone resorption (see **Figure 2**).

Studies have suggested that the expression of RANKL may be increased in the BM of patients with MM. Pearce et al. and Guiliani et al. have both reported increased expression of RANKL by BMSCs from patients with MM; however, no expression was detected in myeloma cells [36,37]. Conversely, Croucher et al. have shown that murine myeloma cells express RANKL on the cell surface, and Sezer et al. have also shown that myeloma cells isolated from the BM of MM patients can express RANKL [38,39]. This raises the possibility that these cells may be able to promote bone resorption directly in a cell contact-dependent manner. Although the reason for the discrepancies between these studies is unclear, the results strongly suggest that RANKL expression may be increased in the local BM microenvironment in patients with MM.

In vitro studies have shown that myeloma cells can decrease the expression of OPG by BMSCs and osteoblasts in a contact-dependent manner [37]. Serum concentrations of OPG are significantly lower in patients with MM than in healthy controls [40]. Furthermore, the ratio of soluble RANKL to OPG is increased in myeloma and correlates with the development of bone disease [41]. It has also been shown that recombinant OPG is able to prevent the development of MM bone disease in the 5T2MM murine model [38]. A recombinant soluble form of RANK has been reported to inhibit the development of osteolytic bone disease in both the 5TGM1 and SCID-human (SCID-hu) murine models of MM [36,42]. Taken together, these data provide strong evidence of a role for the RANKL system in the development of MM bone disease.

Although it is still unclear which of these factors plays the central role in promoting bone resorption in MM, functional studies provide strong evidence of a role for the RANKL system and MIP-1α in this process. However, the possibility that other cytokines and growth factors may also be involved must be considered. For example, studies have shown that a number of factors, including hepatocyte growth factor [43,44] and vascular endothelial growth factor, are produced by myeloma cells and promote bone resorption. However, there are no functional data to support a causal role in MM.

In practice, it is likely that many factors contribute to the regulatory processes responsible for promoting the increase in osteoclastic bone resorption seen in MM. These factors may involve one or two key regulators such as RANKL and/or MIP-1α. Thus, targeting these molecules may provide novel approaches to the management of MM bone disease.

Interdependence between myeloma and bone

Myeloma cells are clearly able to produce factors or express molecules that can promote osteoclast formation and influence bone remodeling. However, the possibility that the environment created by osteoclasts and resorbing bone may be important in promoting the growth and survival of myeloma cells must also be considered. Indeed, many of the cytokines and growth factors that promote the growth and survival of myeloma cells, or modulate their activity, are known to be produced by the cells involved in bone remodeling. For example, IL-6 is produced by human osteoclasts and by primary human osteoblasts; studies have demonstrated that human myeloma cells can induce the production of IL-6 by osteoblasts in a contact-dependent manner [45,46].

Bone itself is also an important source of local growth factors, including transforming growth factor-β and insulin-like growth factor (IGF)-1, amongst others. Myeloma cells express the receptor for IGF-1, and IGF-1 promotes the growth of myeloma cells. IGF-1 is also chemotactic for myeloma cells.

If myeloma cells derive benefit from the environment that is created by resorbing bone, it is anticipated that inhibiting bone resorption and removing this environment would influence myeloma cell growth. There are studies that provide evidence to support this hypothesis. Yacoby et al. have shown that the bisphosphonate zoledronate is able to decrease serum paraprotein concentrations, and promote tumor cell apoptosis in the SCID-hu model of MM [47]. Studies done by Croucher et al. have shown that zoledronate is also able to decrease paraprotein concentrations and reduce tumor burden in the 5T2MM murine model [48]. These studies were associated with a significant increase in survival time in this animal model.

OPG – shown to be effective in inhibiting the development of osteolytic bone disease in the 5T2MM murine model – is also effective at reducing serum paraprotein concentrations in this model [38]. In addition, OPG decreases serum paraprotein concentrations and reduces tumor burden in the 5T33MM murine model, and treatment in this model is associated with a significant increase in survival time [49]. A recombinant soluble form of RANK has also been shown to modulate tumor burden in animal models of MM and hypercalcemia [42,47].

Assessment of MM bone disease

Imaging

A full skeletal survey remains the standard assessment for MM bone disease. It should be performed at diagnosis and at intervals during routine follow-up in order to document the site, size, and progression of lytic bone lesions. Plain X-rays of specific sites are also performed as clinically indicated, eg, to assess new onset of bone pain. The major advantages of plain radiography are speed, universal applicability, and cost. Computed tomography scanning has the advantage of defining smaller lytic lesions than is possible with plain X-rays, and also detects soft-tissue masses associated with bony lesions. Dual-energy X-ray absorptiometry is useful in documenting generalized osteopenia associated with MM.

Magnetic resonance imaging (MRI) is increasingly important in assessing MM. There are certain situations where it is, without doubt, the investigation method of choice. For example, when imaging the spinal cord and cauda equina in the context of new neurologic deficit, it is essential to image the whole vertebral column; this allows visualization of additional, unsuspected lesions, and will permit appropriate planning of treatment with radiation fields adjusted to include all areas requiring therapy. MRI is also extremely useful in the assessment of probable solitary plasmacytoma of bone. When standard investigations have failed to detect any evidence of dissemination beyond an apparently localized tumor, MRI will detect additional sites of disease in up to one third of cases [50]. This will have a major impact on determining appropriate therapy, often indicating the need for additional systemic therapy.

Different patterns of BM infiltration can be appreciated by MRI and are classified as focal, variegated, or diffuse [51]. MRI patterns associated with increasingly heavy marrow infiltration are associated with a poorer outcome and an increased risk of skeletal complications. MRI imaging may be most useful in early stage, asymptomatic disease, where imaging is abnormal in 30%–50% of cases [52]. Patients with an abnormal MRI are at increased risk of disease progression and warrant particularly close follow-up. However, in view of the limited availability and high expense of MRI, it is uncertain whether the technique will become universally applicable.

Biochemical markers of bone resorption

The predominant component of the bone matrix is type I collagen, which is synthesized by osteoblasts. Individual collagen molecules are subsequently covalently linked by pyridinium cross-links in their telopeptide regions. During bone matrix degradation, these cross-linked telopeptides are released and can be detected in the serum and/or urine. Measurement of these telopeptides can be used to monitor the level of matrix degradation. Examples of these telopeptides include the carboxy-terminal telopeptide of type I collagen (ICTP) and the amino-terminal cross-linked telopeptide (NTx). In an analogous manner, the quantity of pyridinium derivatives of type I collagen can be measured in urine as pyridinoline (Pyr) and deoxypyridinoline (dPyr) [53].

In a study of untreated MM patients, ICTP levels correlated with serum β_2-microglobulin; high levels were found in patients with bone pain, lytic lesions, and pathological fractures, and correlated with shorter survival time [54]. Furthermore, urinary Pyr and dPyr levels have been shown to fall following high-dose chemotherapy [55]. These studies indicate that monitoring the levels of biochemical markers of bone resorption may provide valuable information about the extent of bone disease in individual patients, as well as the efficacy of therapeutic interventions in ameliorating ongoing bone degradation.

N-BPs	BPs
Pamidronate	Etidronate
Zoledronate	Clodronate
Risedronate	Tiludronate
Alendronate	
Ibandronate	

Table 1. The nitrogen-containing bisphosphonates (N-BPs) and the non-nitrogen-containing bisphosphonates (BPs).

Bisphosphonate therapy of MM bone disease

Bisphosphonates are the standard therapy for MM. The core structure of bisphosphonate molecules consists of a phosphate–carbon–phosphate (P–C–P) backbone, with differing moieties attached to the R_1 and R_2 side-chains of the central C atom. The R_1 side-chain is usually a hydroxyl group, and this increases the affinity of the molecule for bone. The nature of the R_2 side-chain is variable, but the presence of a nitrogen atom here can be used to classify the bisphosphonates into the nitrogen-containing (the newer therapeutic compounds) and the non-nitrogen-containing (the older therapeutic compounds) bisphosphonates (N-BPs and BPs, respectively) (see **Table 1**).

Mechanism of action

Regardless of the nature of the R_2 side-chain, the P–C–P backbone targets the molecule to calcium-containing bone matrix, which is most exposed at sites of osteoclast activity. Subsequently, the bisphosphonate is liberated from the bone matrix and internalized by osteoclasts, where the drug exerts its antiresorptive activities. It has become evident that BPs and N-BPs possess distinct intracellular activities once internalized [56].

Non-nitrogen-containing bisphosphonates

Within osteoclasts, BPs become incorporated into nonhydrolyzable (AppCp-type) analogs of ATP, which are thought to inhibit a spectrum of intracellular enzymes, resulting in cellular damage [57]. The clodronate metabolite AppCCl2p can be detected in purified osteoclasts from clodronate-treated rabbits; AppCCl2 itself has similar effects, resulting in inhibition of bone resorption and induction of apoptosis [57,58].

Nitrogen-containing bisphosphonates

In vitro, N-BPs have been shown to exhibit a direct proapoptotic effect on myeloma cells [59–61], an effect that also appears to be mediated by inhibiting the pathway responsible for protein prenylation [62]. Several key cellular signaling molecules (eg, the Ras family of GTPases) are only active in their membrane-bound, prenylated forms. Therefore, inhibition of protein prenylation is likely to have significant deleterious effects on cellular function and survival.

N-BPs inhibit farnesyl diphosphate (FPP) synthase and so disrupt the generation of geranylgeranyl diphosphate and FPP itself. The degree to which N-BPs inhibit FPP synthase *in vitro* is paralleled by their *in vivo* antiresorptive activity. The most potent inhibitors of FPP synthase are zoledronate and risedronate [63]. The downstream effects of this inhibition of protein prenylation include the loss of the cell's ruffled border, disruption of the actin cytoskeleton, and induction of osteoclast apoptosis [57]. These effects are thought to be mediated predominantly by the loss of specific geranylgeranylated proteins, such as Rho, Rac, Rab, and cdc42 [64].

Potential additional mechanisms of action for bisphosphonates have been suggested. For instance, N-BPs may have a further indirect effect on myeloma plasma cell survival by inhibiting BMSC production of IL-6 [65]. N-BPs also stimulate peripheral blood γδ T cells *in vitro*. The γδ T cell population represents around 1%–10% of peripheral blood T cells, and these cells recognize antigen in a major histocompatibility complex-unrestricted fashion. Interestingly, their ligands include certain nonpeptide structures that share homology with the P–C–P backbone of bisphosphonates. An attractive hypothesis suggests that bisphosphonates directly stimulate γδ T cells by virtue of this homology. Certainly, the characterization of these previously unrecognized mechanisms of action may facilitate further refinement in drug development. Amongst patients who exhibited an acute phase response after their first infusion of pamidronate, a significant increase in γδ T cell numbers was observed [66]. Furthermore, pamidronate-activated γδ T cells have demonstrated cytotoxicity against lymphoma and myeloma cell lines [67]. Clodronate has been shown to induce γδ T cell proliferation and cytotoxicity in combination with IL-2 and OKT3 (anti-CD3 monoclonal antibody) [68].

The clinical role of bisphosphonate therapy in multiple myeloma

Bisphosphonates have been studied extensively in patients with MM, and the benefits of therapy are well established. The fact that active bone resorption continues even when patients are in the plateau phase of disease indicates that long-term treatment is likely to be appropriate. The increased *in vitro* potency of the newer N-BPs also suggests that these agents may have greater clinical benefit than older BPs.

Clinical trials

Clodronate and other non-nitrogen-containing bisphosphonates

An early study of oral etidronate in MM patients showed that this agent had no demonstrable benefit [69]. Subsequently, two large, randomized, placebo-controlled trials showed clinical benefit from the use of clodronate. The first study recruited 350 newly diagnosed patients who were treated with standard melphalan and prednisone, with or without oral clodronate at a dose of 2.4 g/d [70]. Outcomes were analyzed at 24 months, and a 50% reduction in the rate of progression of osteolytic lesions was observed in the clodronate arm (12% vs. 24%, $P = 0.026$). In addition, there were reductions in the rates of both vertebral and nonvertebral fractures, though the differences were not statistically significant.

The second major clodronate study was part of the UK Medical Research Council (MRC) Myeloma VI trial [71]. Patients with newly diagnosed MM (N = 536) were treated with alkylator-based chemotherapy and randomized to receive placebo or oral clodronate at 1.6 g/d. Patients receiving clodronate experienced significant reductions in the frequency of vertebral fractures (38% vs. 55%; $P = 0.01$) and nonvertebral fractures (5.1% vs. 13.2%; $P = 0.04$), and loss of standing height (2 cm vs. 3.4 cm; $P = 0.01$).

This study made the important observation that patients without overt skeletal disease at diagnosis also benefit from clodronate therapy, indicating that bisphosphonates should be initiated at the same time as chemotherapy, irrespective of the presence of radiologic lesions. Furthermore, a suggestion of prolonged survival in this subgroup of patients prompted a subsequent analysis of the trial after a median follow-up of 8.6 years [72]. Interestingly, clodronate therapy improved survival time for those patients without fractures at diagnosis (59 months vs. 37 months; $P = 0.006$). However, the authors cautioned that these results should not be overinterpreted since this was an unplanned subgroup analysis.

Nitrogen-containing bisphosphonates

Two pivotal papers describe the benefit of pamidronate therapy, given for 9 months and 21 months respectively, to the same cohort of patients [73,74]. In these well-designed studies, 392 patients with stage III MM and at least one lytic lesion were treated with placebo or pamidronate (90 mg/month) intravenously. Patients were receiving either first- or second-line therapy (strata I and II, respectively).

The frequency of skeletal-related events (pathologic fractures, spinal cord compression, hypercalcemia, and the requirement for radiotherapy or surgery) at 9 months was significantly reduced in the pamidronate arm (24% vs. 41%; $P < 0.001$), and this held true for both strata. In addition, the time to first skeletal event was longer (not specified in the paper), while the incidence of hypercalcemia at 3 months (1% vs. 5%) and the degree of bone pain at 9 months (as assessed by scores for bone pain) were lower in the pamidronate arm.

The same group of patients continued to receive their randomized treatment for a further 12 months [74]. When compared with placebo, patients treated with pamidronate experienced a lower mean number of skeletal events per year (1.3 vs. 2.2; $P = 0.008$), and the time to first skeletal event was also prolonged (21 months vs. 10 months; $P < 0.001$). At 21 months, the incidence of skeletal events was reduced in the pamidronate group (38% vs. 51%; $P = 0.15$).

As in the MRC Myeloma VI trial, a survival time advantage was observed in patients on bisphosphonates, but in this trial it was restricted to the more advanced, stratum II patients (median survival time 21 months vs. 14 months; $P = 0.041$). No major toxic events were seen, and, in particular, no adverse effect on renal function was attributed to pamidronate therapy. Although there was a higher incidence of anemia in the pamidronate arm (38% vs. 25%; $P = 0.017$), this did not translate into a greater requirement for transfusion or erythropoietin use.

Pamidronate/zoledronate

Zoledronate is the most potent N-BP currently available, with around 1000-fold greater activity than pamidronate on a weight-for-weight basis. A pooled analysis of two identical randomized studies in patients with hypercalcemia of malignancy (including 8% MM patients) compared pamidronate (90 mg, single dose) with zoledronate (4 mg or 8 mg, single dose). The latter, at either dose, had a higher response rate and a longer interval to relapse [75].

A second dose–response study in 280 patients with lytic lesions (including approximately 40% MM patients) demonstrated that zoledronate at a dose of 2 mg or 4 mg given monthly is as effective as 90 mg pamidronate given monthly in reducing the incidence of skeletal events [76].

A further large, randomized study compared zoledronate (4 mg and 8 mg) with pamidronate (90 mg) in patients with lytic disease resulting from breast cancer (n = 1130) or MM (n = 513) [77]. Among the MM patients, there was no difference between the treatment groups in terms of time to first skeletal event, or incidence of skeletal events at 13 months. There was a slightly higher incidence of renal impairment in patients treated with zoledronate at either dose when the drug was infused over 5 min. However, after the infusion time was prolonged to 15 min, for patients with normal baseline serum creatinine levels, there was no difference in the incidence of renal impairment between patients treated with 4 mg zoledronate and 90 mg pamidronate (9% vs. 8%). The incidence of renal impairment with 8 mg zoledronate given over 15 min was 18% for those patients with normal baseline creatinine levels. Therefore, the risk of renal impairment with zoledronate appears to be related both to dose and to infusion time.

Summary of clinical trials

The results of large, well-designed trials show clear and consistent benefits from the use of both clodronate and pamidronate in MM patients who require therapy. No comparative trials have been, or are likely to be, performed in order to determine the superiority of either of these agents. After reviewing the same clinical trial data, the UK Myeloma Forum recommended long-term pamidronate or clodronate therapy for all patients who require treatment for MM (see **Table 2**) [78]. The UK Myeloma Forum Guidelines have subsequently been revised and amended (March 2003; see www.ukmf.org.uk), and 4 mg zoledronate monthly is stated as an alternative to pamidronate, though caution is advised in the setting of renal failure, and a 15 min infusion is recommended. An expert panel convened by the American Society of Clinical Oncology (ASCO) recommends pamidronate (or zoledronate) for all patients with lytic disease (see **Table 3**) [79]. The panel did not recommend the use of clodronate due to its current unavailability in the USA, and also because of perceived deficiencies in the methodological

Recommendation	Grade of recommendation	Level of evidence
Long-term bisphosphonate therapy should be used in all MM patients who need treatment (whether bone lesions are evident or not).	A[1]	Ib[2]
Administration of oral clodronate (1600 mg/d) or intravenous pamidronate is effective for MM patients.	A	Ib
Intravenous zoledronate 4 mg monthly is equivalent to pamidronate 90 mg monthly and may be used in preference to pamidronate.	A	Ib
Etidronate should be avoided in the treatment of MM patients.	A	Ib
Caution is required when administering bisphosphonates to patients with moderate to severe renal failure.	A	Ib

Table 2. UK Myeloma Forum Guidelines on the Diagnosis and Management of Multiple Myeloma [78]. Recommendations for the use of bisphosphonates. MM: multiple myeloma. The guideline for zoledronate was added as a revision in December 2002 and amended in March 2003 (see: www.ukmf.org.uk).

[1]Grade A is defined as: a recommendation based on at least one randomized, controlled trial of good quality and consistency addressing a specific recommendation.

[2]Level Ib is defined as: evidence obtained from at least one randomized, controlled trial.

design of the clodronate studies. Since renal complications appear to be related to both the dose and speed of infusion of zoledronate, the ASCO expert panel concluded that zoledronate should be infused at a dose of 4 mg over a period of at least 15 min. The benefits of a reduced infusion time for zoledronate must be weighed against the greater cost of the drug.

Recommendation	Grade of recommendation	Level of evidence
MM patients with lytic disease should receive intravenous pamidronate (90 mg) or zoledronate (4 mg) every 3–4 weeks.	B[1]	II[4]
In MM patients with creatinine levels <265 μmol/L, the standard dose and infusion times can be used for pamidronate or zoledronate.	D[3]	V[6]
Infusion times of <2 h should be avoided with pamidronate.		
Infusion times of <15 min should be avoided with zoledronate.		
Regular monitoring of renal function should be carried out in MM patients with albuminuria and azotemia.		
Intravenous administration of pamidronate or zoledronate should continue until there is a substantial decline in the patient's performance score.	Panel consensus	N/A
Use intravenous bisphosphonate treatment in MM patients with osteopenia but no radiographic evidence of lytic bone disease.	Panel consensus	N/A
Do not use bisphosphonates to treat patients with SPB, SM, or IMM. (Awaiting trials.)	Panel consensus	N/A
Do not use bisphosphonates to treat patients with MGUS. (Awaiting trials.)	Panel consensus	N/A
The use of biochemical markers of bone metabolism to monitor bisphosphonate use is not needed in routine cases.	C[2]	III[5]
Intravenous pamidronate or zoledronate should be used in patients with pain caused by osteolytic disease adjunctive to radiotherapy, analgesics, or surgery to stabilize fractures/impending fractures.	B	II

Table 3. American Society of Clinical Oncology clinical practice guidelines for the role of bisphosphonates in multiple myeloma (MM) [79]. IMM = indolent multiple myeloma; MGUS: monoclonal gammopathy of undetermined significance; SM: smoldering myeloma; SPB: solitary plasmacytoma of bone. [1]Grade B defined as: evidence of types II, III, or IV, and findings generally consistent. [2]Grade C defined as: evidence of types II, III, or IV, but findings inconsistent. [3]Grade D defined as: little or no systematic empirical evidence. [4]Level II defined as: evidence from at least one well-designed experimental study. Randomized trials with high false-positive and/or -negative errors (low power). [5]Level III defined as: evidence obtained from well-designed, quasi-experimental studies such as nonrandomized, controlled single-group, pre-post, cohort, time, or matched case-control series. [6]Level V defined as: evidence from case reports and clinical examples.

Non-bisphosphonate treatment of MM bone disease

The use of bisphosphonate therapy is well established and represents a major advance in the treatment of MM. However, additional therapies are available.

Cytotoxic chemotherapy

It is clear that chemotherapy will have an impact on MM bone disease. By killing malignant plasma cells, chemotherapy interrupts the mutually stimulatory interactions between plasma cells and the BM microenvironment that result in bone degradation. Direct evidence for this is provided by observations that high-dose chemotherapy reduces the levels of biochemical markers of bone resorption [55], and that lytic lesions heal after successful treatment.

Radiotherapy

Since MM is relatively sensitive to radiotherapy, this is an appropriate form of local treatment for painful lytic lesions, for vertebral disease threatening or resulting in cord or root compression, or as an adjunctive treatment for pathologic fractures.

Surgery

Surgery is an important component in the management of impending or completed pathologic fractures. Intramedullary nails are often inserted into long bones with large lytic lesions that threaten pathologic fracture. Surgery is often appropriate when there is spinal cord compression or instability, and is then combined with local radiotherapy. Total hip replacement should be considered for patients with acetabular or periarticular pelvic disease [80].

A relatively new approach is the use of percutaneous vertebroplasty, in which bone cement is injected directly into vertebral bodies with the aim of improving pain and preventing vertebral collapse [81]. Although this technique can provide rapid pain relief, it is not free from side effects (eg, radiculopathy due to leakage of cement) and its place in the management of vertebral disease remains uncertain. In order to overcome the problems associated with vertebroplasty, a procedure known as kyphoplasty has been developed. This involves the initial insertion of an inflatable bone tamp into the fractured vertebral body, inflation of the balloon to elevate the endplates, and subsequent deflation and withdrawal, thus leaving a cavity within the vertebral body itself. This cavity is then filled with bone cement. An initial study involving this procedure [82] has reported a 34% average correction of height loss, along with significant improvements in scores for bodily pain as well as physical and social functioning. Asymptomatic cement leakage occurred in 4% of procedures. These encouraging findings may well lead to the more widespread use of this technique in patients with MM.

Conclusions and future directions

Bone disease is a major factor in the morbidity and mortality of patients with MM. The mechanisms of bone resorption are complex, multifactorial, and, to a great extent, result from mutually stimulatory interactions between tumor cells and various components of the BM microenvironment itself. A number of autocrine, paracrine, and cell–cell adhesive mechanisms are critically involved in these interactions, and establish a vicious cycle whereby bone resorption is amplified at the same time that tumor cell survival and proliferation are enhanced.

The clinical utility of the bisphosphonates is now well established. These agents directly inhibit bone resorption and result in osteoclast apoptosis. In addition, there is some *in vitro* evidence to suggest that these agents possess direct antitumor properties in their own right.

As the complex mechanisms of bone resorption are elucidated with greater clarity, new targets for therapeutic intervention are being identified. Indeed, early preclinical studies of recombinant

OPG and the recombinant soluble form of the receptor RANK (RANK-Fc) show distinct promise [38,47,83,84]. The emergence of MIP-1α as a mediator of MM bone disease presents another potential target for intervention. As greater understanding of the pathophysiology of MM bone disease evolves, it is hoped that significant improvements in treatment can be devised that will have a major impact on the quality of life of patients suffering from this complex, progressive malignancy.

References

1. Lahtinen R, Laakso M, Palva I et al. Randomised, placebo-controlled multicentre trial of clodronate in multiple myeloma. Finnish Leukaemia Group. *Lancet* 1992;340:1049–52.
2. Kanis JA, McCloskey EV. Disorders of calcium and skeletal metabolism. In: Malpas JS, Bersagel DE, Kyle RA, editors. *Myeloma: Biology and Management*. New York, NY: Oxford University Press, 1997.
3. Valentin-Opran A, Charhon SA, Meunier PJ et al. Quantitative histology of myeloma-induced bone changes. *Br J Haematol* 1982;52:601–10.
4. Bataille R, Chappard D, Marcelli C et al. Recruitment of new osteoblasts and osteoclasts is the earliest critical event in the pathogenesis of human multiple myeloma. *J Clin Invest* 1991;88:62–6.
5. Taube T, Beneton MN, McCloskey EV et al. Abnormal bone remodelling in patients with myelomatosis and normal biochemical indices of bone resorption. *Eur J Hematol* 1992;49:192–8.
6. Roux C, Ravaud P, Cohen-Solal M et al. Biologic, histologic and densitometric effects of oral risedronate on bone in patients with multiple myeloma. *Bone* 1994;15:41–9.
7. Bataille R, Chappard D, Basle M. Quantifiable excess of bone resorption in monoclonal gammopathy is an early symptom of malignancy: a prospective study of 87 bone biopsies. *Blood* 1996;87:4762–9.
8. Bataille R, Chappard D, Basle MF. Excessive bone resorption in human plasmacytomas: direct induction by tumour cells *in vivo*. *Br J Haematol* 1995;90:721–4.
9. Mundy GR, Luben RA, Raisz LG et al. Bone-resorbing activity in supernatants from lymphoid cell lines. *N Engl J Med* 1974;290:867–71.
10. Mundy GR, Raisz LG, Cooper RA et al. Evidence for the secretion of an osteoclast stimulating factor in myeloma. *N Engl J Med* 1974;291:1041–6.
11. Lichtenstein A, Berenson J, Norman D et al. Production of cytokines by bone marrow cells obtained from patients with multiple myeloma. *Blood* 1989;74:1266–73.
12. Cozzolino F, Torcia M, Aldinucci D et al. Production of interleukin-1 by bone marrow myeloma cells. *Blood* 1989;74:380–7.
13. Kawano M, Yamamoto I, Iwato K et al. Interleukin-1 beta rather than lymphotoxin as the major bone resorbing activity in human multiple myeloma. *Blood* 1989;73:1646–9.
14. Yamamoto I, Kawano M, Sone T et al. Production of interleukin-1 beta, a potent bone resorbing cytokine, by human myeloma cells. *Cancer Res* 1989;49:4242–6.
15. Bakkus MHC, Bakel-Van Peer KMJ et al. Detection of interleukin-1β and interleukin-6 in human multiple myeloma by fluorescent in situ hybridisation. *Leuk Lymphoma* 1991;4:389–95.

16. Sati HAI, Greaves M, Apperley JF et al. Expression of interleukin-1beta and tumour necrosis factor-alpha in plasma cells from patients with multiple myeloma. *Br J Haematol* 1996;104:350–7.
17. Borset M, Helseth E, Naume B et al. Lack of IL-1 secretion from human myeloma cells highly purified by immunomagnetic separation. *Br J Haematol* 1993;85:446–51.
18. Garrett IR, Durie BG, Nedwin GE et al. Production of lymphotoxin, a bone resorbing cytokine, by cultured human myeloma cells. *N Engl J Med* 1987;317:526–32.
19. Bataille R, Klein B, Jourdan M et al. Spontaneous secretion of tumor necrosis factor-beta by human myeloma cell lines. *Cancer* 1989;63:877–80.
20. Kawano M, Hirano T, Matsuda T et al. Autocrine generation and requirement of BSF-2/IL-6 for human multiple myelomas. *Nature* 1988;332:83–5.
21. Klein B, Zhang XG, Lu ZY et al. Interleukin-6 in human multiple myeloma. *Blood* 1995;85:863–72.
22. Anderson KC, Jones RC, Morimoto C et al. Response patterns of purified myeloma cells to hematopoietic growth factors. *Blood* 1989;73:1915–24.
23. Westendorf JF, Ahmann GJ, Armitage RJ et al. CD40 expression in malignant plasma cells. Role in stimulation of autocrine IL-6 secretion by a human myeloma cell line. *J Immunol* 1994;152:117–28.
24. Urashima M, Chauhan D, Uchiyama H et al. CD40 ligand triggered interleukin-6 secretion in multiple myeloma. *Blood* 1995;85:1903–12.
25. Sati HI, Apperley JF, Greaves M et al. Interleukin-6 is expressed by plasma cells from patients with multiple myeloma and monoclonal gammopathy of undetermined significance. *Br J Haematol* 1998;101:287–95.
26. Uchiyama H, Barut BA, Mohrbacher AF et al. Adhesion of human myeloma-derived cell lines to bone marrow stromal cells stimulates interleukin-6 secretion. *Blood* 1993;82:3712–20.
27. Lokhorst HM, Lamme T, de Smet M et al. Primary tumor cells of myeloma patients induce interleukin-6 secretion in long-term bone marrow cultures. *Blood* 1994;84:2269–77.
28. Lowik CW, van der Pluijm G, Bloys H et al. Parathyroid hormone (PTH) and PTH-like protein (PLP) stimulate interleukin-6 production by osteogenic cells: a possible role of interleukin-6 in osteoclasteogenesis. *Biochem Biophys Res Commun* 1989;162:1546–52.
29. Roodman GD. Interleukin-6: an osteotropic factor? *J Bone Miner Res* 1992;7:475–8.
30. Choi SJ, Cruz JC, Craig F at al. Macrophage inflammatory protein 1-alpha is a potential osteoclast stimulatory factor in multiple myeloma. *Blood* 2000;96:671–75.
31. Choi SJ, Oba Y, Gazitt Y et al. Antisense inhibition of macrophage inflammatory protein 1-alpha blocks bone destruction in a model of myeloma bone disease. *J Clin Invest* 2001;108:1833–41.
32. Oyajobi BO, Franchin G, Williams PJ et al. Dual effects of macrophage inflammatory protein-1{alpha} on osteolysis and tumor burden in the murine 5TGM1 model of myeloma bone disease. *Blood* 2003;Mar 20 [Epub ahead of print].
33. Anderson DM, Maraskovsky E, Billingsley WL et al. A homologue of the TNF receptor and its ligand enhance T-cell growth and dendritic cell function. *Nature* 1997;390:175–9.
34. Kong YY, Yoshida H, Sarosi I et al. OPGL is a key regulator of osteoclastogenesis, lymphocyte development and lymph-node organogenesis. *Nature* 1999;397:315–23.
35. Simonet WS, Lacey DL, Dunstan CR et al. Osteoprotegerin: a novel secreted protein involved in the regulation of bone density. *Cell* 1997;89:309–19.
36. Pearce RN, Sordillo EM, Yaccoby S et al. Multiple myeloma disrupts the TRANCE/osteoprotegerin cytokine axis to trigger bone destruction and promote tumor progression. *Proc Nat Acad Sci USA* 2001;98:11581–6.

37. Giuliani N, Bataille R, Mancini C et al. Myeloma cells induce imbalance in the osteoprotegerin/osteoprotegerin ligand system in the human bone marrow environment. *Blood* 2001;98:3527–33.
38. Croucher PI, Shipman CM, Lippitt J et al. Osteoprotegerin inhibits the development of osteolytic bone disease in multiple myeloma. *Blood* 2001;98:3534–40.
39. Sezer O, Heider U, Jakob C et al. Human bone marrow myeloma cells express RANKL. *J Clin Oncol* 2002;20:353–4.
40. Seidel C, Hjertner O, Abildgaard N et al. Serum osteoprotegerin levels are reduced in patients with multiple myeloma with bone disease. *Blood* 2001;98:2269–71.
41. Terpos E, Szydlo R, Apperley JF et al. Soluble receptor activator of nuclear factor {kappa}B ligand (RANKL)/osteoprotegerin (OPG) ratio predicts survival in multiple myeloma. Proposal for a novel prognostic index. *Blood* 2003;Apr 10 [Epub ahead of print].
42. Oyajobi BO, Garrett IR et al. A soluble murine receptor activator of NF-kB-human immunoglobulin fusion protein (RANK.Fc) inhibits bone resorption in a murine model of human multiple myeloma bone disease. *J Bone Min Res* 2000;15:S176 (Abstr.).
43. Borset M, Hjorth-Hansen H, Seidel C et al. Hepatocyte growth factor and its receptor c-met in multiple myeloma. *Blood* 1996;88:3998–4004.
44. Borset M, Lien E, Espevik T et al. Concomitant expression of hepatocyte growth factor/scatter factor and the receptor c-MET in human myeloma cell lines. *J Biol Chem* 1996;271:24655–61.
45. Barille S, Collette M, Bataille R et al. Myeloma cells upregulate interleukin-6 secretion in osteoblastic cells through cell-to-cell contact but downregulate osteocalcin. *Blood* 1995;86:3151–9.
46. Karadag A, Oyajobi BO, Apperley JF et al. Human myeloma cells promote the production of interleukin 6 by primary human osteoblasts. *Br J Haematol* 2000;108:383–90.
47. Yaccoby S, Pearse RN, Johnson CL et al. Myeloma interacts with the bone marrow microenvironment to induce osteoclastogenesis and is dependent on osteoclast activity. *Br J Haematol* 2002;116:278–90.
48. Croucher PI, De Hendrik R, Perry MJ et al. Zoledronic acid treatment of 5T2MM-bearing mice inhibits the development of myeloma bone disease: evidence for decreased osteolysis, tumor burden and angiogenesis, and increased survival. *J Bone Miner Res* 2003;18:482–92.
49. Vanderkerken K, Asosingh K, Van Camp B et al. Recombinant osteoprotegerin decreases tumor burden and increases survival in a murine model of multiple myeloma. *Cancer Res* 2003;63:287–89.
50. Moulopoulos LA, Dimopoulos MA, Weber D et al. Magnetic resonance imaging in the staging of solitary plasmacytoma of bone. *J Clin Oncol* 1993;11:1311–5.
51. Moulopoulos LA, Dimopoulos MA. Magnetic resonance imaging of the bone marrow in hematological malignancies. *Blood* 1997;90:2127–47.
52. Moulopoulos LA, Dimopoulos MA, Smith TL et al. Prognostic significance of magnetic resonance imaging in patients with asymptomatic multiple myeloma. *J Clin Oncol* 1995;13:251–6.
53. Callander NS, Roodman GD. Myeloma bone disease. *Semin Hematol* 2001;38:276–85.
54. Fonseca R, Trendle MC, Leong T et al. Prognostic value of serum markers of bone metabolism in untreated multiple myeloma patients. *Br J Haematol* 2000;109:24–9.
55. Clark RE, Flory AJ, Ion EM et al. Biochemical markers of bone turnover following high-dose chemotherapy and autografting in multiple myeloma. *Blood* 2000;96:2697–702.
56. Russel RG, Rogers MJ. Bisphosphonates: from the laboratory to the clinic and back again. *Bone* 1999;25:97–106.

57. Rogers MJ, Gordon S, Benford HL et al. Cellular and molecular mechanisms of action of bisphosphonates. *Cancer* 2000;88(12 Suppl.):2961–78.
58. Frith JC, Monkkonen J, Auriola S et al. The molecular mechanism of action of the antiresorptive and anti-inflammatory drug clodronate: evidence for the formation *in vivo* of a metabolite that inhibits bone resorption and causes osteoclast and macrophage apoptosis. *Arthritis Rheum* 2001;44:2201–10.
59. Shipman CM, Rogers MJ, Apperley JF et al. Bisphosphonates induce apoptosis in human myeloma cell lines: a novel anti-tumour activity. *Br J Haematol* 1997;98:665–72.
60. Tassone P, Forciniti S, Galea E et al. Growth inhibition and synergistic induction of apoptosis by zoledronate and dexamethasone in human myeloma cell lines. *Leukemia* 2000;14:841–4.
61. Aparicio A, Gardner A, Tu Y et al. *In vitro* cytoreductive effects on multiple myeloma cells induced by bisphosphonates. *Leukemia* 1998;12:220–9.
62. Shipman M, Croucher PI, Russell RGG et al. The bisphosphonate YM175 causes apoptosis of human myeloma cells *in vitro* by inhibiting the mevalonate pathway. *Cancer Res* 1998;58:5294–7.
63. Dunford JE, Thompson K, Coxon FP et al. Structure-activity relationships for inhibition of farnesyl diphosphate synthase *in vitro* and inhibition of bone resorption *in vivo* by nitrogen-containing bisphosphonates. *J Pharmacol Exp Ther* 2001;296:235–42.
64. Coxon FP, Helfrich MH, Van't Hof R et al. Protein geranylgeranylation is required for osteoclast formation, function, and survival: inhibition by bisphosphonates and GGTI-298. *J Bone Miner Res* 2000;15:1467–76.
65. Derenne S, Amiot M, Barille S et al. Zoledronate is a potent inhibitor of myeloma cell growth and secretion of IL-6 and MMP-1 by the tumoral environment. *J Bone Miner Res* 1999;14:2048–56.
66. Kunzmann V, Bauer E, Wilhelm M. Gamma/delta T-cell stimulation by pamidronate. *N Engl J Med* 1999;340:737–8 (letter).
67. Kunzmann V, Bauer E, Feurle J et al. Stimulation of gammadelta T cells by aminobisphosphonates and induction of antiplasma cell activity in multiple myeloma. *Blood* 2000;96:384–92.
68. Schilbach K, Geiselhart A, Handgretinger R. Induction of proliferation and augmented cytotoxicity of gammadelta T lymphocytes by bisphosphonate clodronate. *Blood* 2001;97:2917–8 (letter).
69. Belch AR, Bergsagel DE, Wilson K et al. Effect of daily etidronate on the osteolysis of multiple myeloma. *J Clin Oncol* 1991;9:1397–402.
70. Lahtinen R, Laakso M, Palva I et al. Randomised, placebo-controlled multicentre trial of clodronate in multiple myeloma. Finnish Leukemia Group. *Lancet* 1992;340:1049–52.
71. McCloskey EV, MacLennan IC, Drayson MT et al. A randomised trial of the effect of clodronate on skeletal morbidity in multiple myeloma. *Br J Haematol* 1998;100:317–25.
72. McCloskey EV, Dunn JA, Kanis JA et al. Long-term follow-up of a prospective, double-blind, placebo-controlled randomized trial of clodronate in multiple myeloma. *Br J Haematol* 2001;113:1035–43.
73. Berenson JR, Lichtenstein A, Porter L et al. Efficacy of pamidronate in reducing skeletal events in patients with advanced multiple myeloma. Myeloma Aredia Study Group. *N Engl J Med* 1996;334:488–93.
74. Berenson JR, Lichtenstein A, Porter L et al. Long-term pamidronate treatment of advanced multiple myeloma patients reduces skeletal events. *J Clin Oncol* 1998;16:593–602.
75. Major P, Lortholary A, Hon J et al. Zoledronic acid is superior to pamidronate in the treatment of hypercalcaemia of malignancy: a pooled analysis of two randomised, controlled clinical trials. *J Clin Oncol* 2001;19:558–67.

76. Berenson JR, Rosen LS, Howell A et al. Zoledronic acid reduces skeletal-related events in patients with osteolytic metastases. *Cancer* 2001;91:1191–200.
77. Rosen LS, Gordon D, Kaminski M et al. Zoledronic acid versus pamidronate in the treatment of skeletal metastases in patients with breast cancer or osteolytic lesions of multiple myeloma: a phase III, double-blind, comparative trial. *Cancer J* 2001;7:377–87.
78. Guidelines Committee of the UK Myeloma Forum on behalf of the UK Myeloma Forum. British Committee for Standards in Haematology. Guideline: Diagnosis and management of multiple myeloma. *Br J Haematol* 2001;115:522–40.
79. Berenson JR, Hillner BE, Kyle RA et al. American Society of Clinical Oncology clinical practice guidelines: the role of bisphosphonates in multiple myeloma. *J Clin Oncol* 2002;20:3719–36.
80. Papagelopoulos PJ, Galanis EC, Greipp PR et al. Prosthetic hip replacement for pathologic or impending pathologic fractures in myeloma. *Clin Orthop* 1997;341:192–205.
81. Martin JB, Jean B, Sugiu K et al. Vertebroplasty: clinical experience and follow-up results. *Bone* 1999;25(2 Suppl.):11S–15S.
82. Dudeney S, Lieberman IH, Reinhardt M-K et al. Kyphoplasty in the treatment of osteolytic vertebral compression fractures as a result of multiple myeloma. *J Clin Oncol* 2002;20:2382–7.
83. Griepp P et al. A single subcutaneous dose of an osteoprotegerin (OPG) construct (AMGN-0007) causes a profound and sustained decrease of bone resorption comparable to standard intravenous bisphosphonate in patients with multiple myeloma. *Blood* 1998;92(Suppl. 1):A3227.
84. Oyajobi BO, Anderson DM, Traianedes K et al. Therapeutic efficacy of a soluble receptor activator of nuclear factor kappaB-IgG Fc fusion protein in suppressing bone resorption and hypercalcemia in a model of humoral hypercalcemia of malignancy. *Cancer Res* 2001;61:2572–8.

7

Approach to management and supportive care

S Vincent Rajkumar & Robert A Kyle

Introduction

Current therapy for multiple myeloma (MM) is not curative. However, over the last few years, substantial advances have been made in the management of this disease. These include the use of autologous stem cell transplantation (ASCT), thalidomide, bisphosphonates, and bortezomib [1]. A number of key clinical trials have been completed, and the results of these strategies are now available. This chapter summarizes recent advances and provides an overall approach to the management of MM. The various supportive care options for patients with MM are also reviewed.

Diagnosis of multiple myeloma

The initial step in the management of MM involves a critical diagnostic evaluation to differentiate the disease from other closely related disorders, such as monoclonal gammopathy of undetermined significance (MGUS), smoldering (asymptomatic) myeloma (SM), solitary plasmacytoma, and primary amyloidosis (AL) (see **Figure 1**) [2].

Monoclonal gammopathy of undetermined significance

Patients with MGUS are asymptomatic and do not require therapy. However, they need indefinite follow-up because symptomatic MM or related malignancy develops at a rate of approximately 1% of MGUS patients per year [3]. The size of the monoclonal (M) protein concentration is the most important prognostic factor

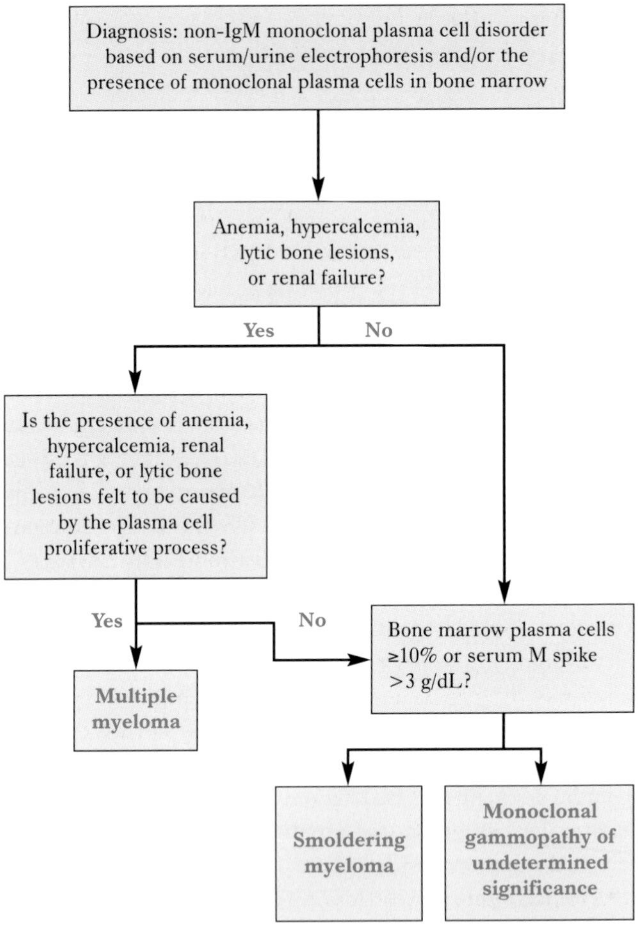

- Patients with plasma cell disorders described above who have symptoms consistent with amyloidosis should have Congo Red staining done for the presence of amyloid on the bone marrow/fat aspirate and, if needed, on the sample of tissue involved.
- Patients with a single bony or extramedullary plasmacytoma and bone marrow <10% plasma cells are considered to have "solitary plasmacytoma".

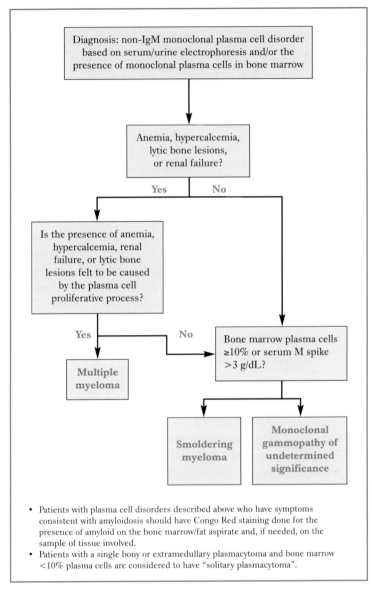

Figure 1. Differential diagnosis of monoclonal gammopathy of undetermined significance, solitary plasmacytoma, multiple myeloma, smoldering myeloma, and primary amyloidosis. Ig: immunoglobulin.

in predicting the rate of progression [4]. Patients with immunoglobulin (Ig)M MGUS have a higher risk of progression than those with IgA or IgG M proteins. Cesana and colleagues have shown that a bone marrow plasma cell percentage of 6%–9% carries twice the risk of progression compared with marrow involvement that is ≤5% [5]. There are conflicting reports regarding the relationship of disease progression to reduced uninvolved Ig levels and the presence of urinary M proteins [4,5]. Clearly, additional laboratory predictors of progression from MGUS to myeloma are necessary.

At the Mayo Clinic (Rochester, MN, USA), the serum M protein level is rechecked at 6 months; if stable, it is then checked annually thereafter.

Smoldering (asymptomatic) myeloma

Patients with SM, like those with MGUS, are also asymptomatic, but have a much higher risk of progression to MM. The median time to progression is 1–2 years [6], though some patients can remain stable without therapy for several years [7]. SM patients with abnormal results from peripheral blood monoclonal plasma cell studies – defined as an increase in the number or proliferative rate of circulating plasma cells as detected by immunofluorescent assays – are at higher risk for earlier progression to MM [8]. In a study of 57 patients, Witzig et al. found that the median time to progression was 9 months for those with abnormal circulating plasma cell values versus 30 months for those with normal values ($P<0.01$) [8]. Other risk factors that predict progression of SM to MM include the presence of occult lytic lesions on magnetic resonance imaging [9–11] and elevated bone marrow plasma cell labeling index results [12]. Patients with high serum M protein values (>3 g/dL) and those with IgA-type M protein are also at higher risk of progression [9].

Due to the toxicity of alkylator- or steroid-based chemotherapy, the lack of evidence of benefit, and the fact that some patients can remain progression free for several years without therapy, the current standard of care in SM is close observation without drug therapy [6,7,13]. However, selected patients can be considered for appropriate clinical trials that evaluate novel, investigational, low-toxicity therapy. Thalidomide has shown some promise in early studies [14–17]. The response rate in 31 patients with early-stage MM was 34%, with a progression-free survival rate at 2 years of 63% [17]. Similarly, bisphosphonates such as pamidronate and zoledronate can prevent or delay bone lesions in patients with MM [18–21], and also have the potential to be effective in SM. However, given the toxicity of long-term therapy, randomized trials will be necessary to establish the role of thalidomide and bisphosphonates in SM. A randomized trial comparing thalidomide plus zoledronate versus zoledronate alone in SM is ongoing at the Mayo Clinic.

Solitary plasmacytoma

Patients with solitary plasmacytoma present with the following indications [22]:

- a single plasmacytoma (bony or extramedullary)
- M protein (may or may not be present)
- bone marrow that is not consistent with MM (ie, ≤10% plasma cells)
- no evidence of other bone or extramedullary lesions
- no anemia, renal failure, or hypercalcemia

For patients with solitary plasmacytoma, standard treatment consists of tumor radiation therapy (40–45 Gy) to the involved area followed by close observation [22,23]. Chemotherapy is not indicated. The 10-year disease-free survival rate following radiation therapy is approximately 25%–45% [22]. However, many patients progress to overt MM, with a median time to progression of approximately 3 years. The risk of progression is increased significantly if patients have residual M protein after definitive radiation therapy [24]. Recently, the presence of increased angiogenesis in the plasmacytoma has been identified as another significant risk factor for progression to MM [25].

Primary amyloidosis

Primary AL is a rare plasma cell proliferative condition in which insoluble monoclonal light-chain Ig fragments are deposited as a β-pleated fibrillar substance in various organs [26,27]. The most common clinical presentations include nephrotic syndrome, restrictive cardiomyopathy, peripheral neuropathy, macroglossia, and hepatomegaly. Patients may have one or more organs involved at presentation, and the number of organs involved is a key prognostic factor for the disease. The presence of cardiac AL is also an adverse prognostic factor.

The diagnosis of primary AL requires two steps. First, is histologic proof of amyloid. This is best done by biopsy of the abdominal fat (fat aspirate), bone marrow, and, if needed, the organ or tissue suspected of involvement. The diagnosis is based on Congo Red staining, with a characteristic apple-green birefringence seen under polarized light.

The second step is evidence that the AL is of the light-chain type (primary AL), since forms of amyloid unrelated to plasma cell disorders do exist. These include senile amyloid due to unmutated transthyretin, hereditary amyloid due to mutated transthyretin, and secondary amyloid (in patients with chronic inflammation) due to serum amyloid A protein. Evidence that AL is of the light-chain type is best done by testing for the presence of serum and urine M proteins and/or monoclonal bone marrow plasma cells. Patients with a compatible clinical picture with evidence of a monoclonal plasma cell disorder and histologic proof of amyloid are empirically considered to have primary AL. In difficult cases, staining of the amyloid tissue for κ/λ light chains can help differentiate primary AL from other forms of AL.

The current standard therapy for primary AL is oral melphalan/prednisone [25]. An alternative is high-dose corticosteroids. Colchicine does not seem to be of benefit [28]. High-dose chemotherapy followed by stem cell transplantation provides superior response rates, but it should still be considered investigational [29] since transplantation in primary AL is associated with increased morbidity and mortality over MM.

The treatment of multiple myeloma

Approach to therapy

Patients who are asymptomatic, with only mild anemia or small lytic lesions on skeletal survey (eg, patients with indolent MM), can be monitored without therapy in a similar way to patients with SM. Such patients may also benefit from bisphosphonate therapy with either pamidronate or zoledronate, particularly if they have lytic lesions or osteoporosis.

Therapy is indicated for symptomatic patients with MM. A schematic approach to the management of patients with newly diagnosed MM is shown in **Figure 2** [1]. Once it is decided that therapy is indicated, the physician needs to consider whether the patient is a candidate for ASCT, since the optimal survival time is achieved with this strategy [30,31]. Enrollment on appropriate clinical trials must be considered for all patients. Outside the setting of a clinical trial, patients who are not candidates for ASCT – due to either advanced age, poor performance status, significant renal failure, or comorbidity – are best treated with conventional-dose, alkylator-based chemotherapy with melphalan and prednisone. Patients who are eligible for transplantation are treated with early or delayed ASCT.

Conventional-dose chemotherapy: melphalan and prednisone

Melphalan plus prednisone remains the principal therapy for patients who are not transplant candidates. The overall response rate with this regimen is approximately 50% [32].

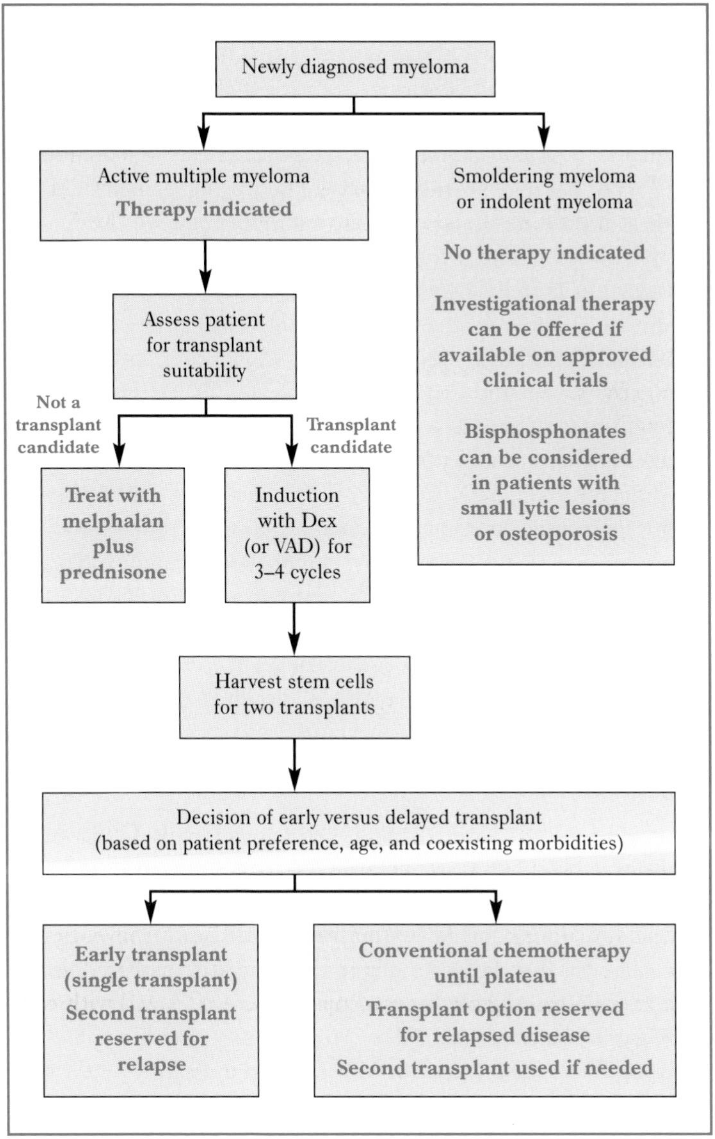

Figure 2. Suggested approach to the treatment of newly diagnosed multiple myeloma. Modified with permission from Rajkumar SV, Kyle RA [1]. Dex: dexamethasone; VAD: vincristine, doxorubicin, and dexamethasone.

The complete remission (CR) rate is less than 10% and the median survival time is about 3 years [33]. The 5-year survival rate is approximately 25% [32].

Melphalan is usually administered orally at a dose of 0.15 mg/kg/d for 7 days; during the same 7 days, prednisone is administered orally at a dose of 60 mg/d. This treatment regimen is repeated every 6 weeks. The white blood cell and platelet counts are typically measured 3 weeks and 6 weeks after the start of treatment. Based on these counts, the dose of melphalan in subsequent cycles is adjusted to produce mild cytopenia at mid-cycle to ensure that the dose of melphalan is adequate. Patients are treated in this manner for 1 year, or for up to 6 months after a plateau phase has been achieved.

More aggressive combination chemotherapy regimens such as VBMCP (vincristine, carmustine, melphalan, cyclophosphamide, prednisone) result in superior response rates (60%–70%), but have no substantial survival benefit over melphalan plus prednisone [32,34,35]. The addition of interferon (IFN)-α (usual dose: 3 million units, three times weekly) to initial therapy produces slightly better response rates, but no clinically beneficial improvement in survival [36].

Autologous stem cell transplantation (also see Chapter 5)

High-dose chemotherapy followed by ASCT is not curative in MM, but it improves the response rate and survival time [37–40]. Overall response rates with transplant are approximately 75%–90% [33,34] and CR rates range from 20% to 40% [30,38]. The French group Intergroupe Francophone du Myelome (IFM) conducted a randomized trial of 200 previously untreated patients. The overall survival time with ASCT was significantly better than with conventional-dose chemotherapy, with 5-year survival rates of 52% and 12%, respectively [30]. A recent study by Child and colleagues from the UK Medical Research Council (MRC) Adult Leukaemia Working Party confirmed the superiority of ASCT over conventional chemotherapy [31]. Although preliminary data from a recent randomized trial by the Spanish Cooperative group have brought into question the magnitude of the survival benefit achieved with transplantation [41], ASCT remains the current standard of care for eligible patients. One difference between the Spanish trial and those by the French and MRC groups is that the only patients who were randomized in the Spanish trial were those who responded to induction therapy.

Age >65 years is not, on its own, a contraindication for transplantation [42]. Such patients are candidates for transplantation if they have good functional status and limited comorbidity.

Timing of transplantation

ASCT can be delayed until relapse, without compromising survival, if hematopoietic stem cells are harvested and cryopreserved prior to alkylator therapy. Data from two French randomized trials comparing early versus delayed transplantation indicate that there is no significant difference in overall survival time between the two procedures [43–45]. However, there was a significant advantage in quality of life with early ASCT. Data from another large multicenter randomized trial addressing this issue have recently completed accrual in the US and are awaiting analysis. At present, the choice between the two options is based mainly on patient preference, though other coexisting medical problems and risk factors may play a role in the decision-making process.

Pretransplant induction regimen

Infusional vincristine, doxorubicin, and pulsed dexamethasone (VAD) is considered by many investigators to be the standard pretransplant induction therapy [46,47]. However, VAD is cumbersome and is associated with substantial toxicity. Lack of response to VAD, such as that observed in patients with primary refractory MM, is not a predictor of poor survival time following transplantation, and patients are treated with transplantation regardless of their response to VAD [48,49].

Dexamethasone accounts for almost 80% of the activity of VAD. A single-institution study observed response rates of 43% with dexamethasone alone and 55% with VAD [50,46]. Although the response rate is lower with dexamethasone alone, there is no effect on overall survival [50]. Similarly, there is no difference in engraftment or stem cell collection with either dexamethasone alone or VAD [51]. Therefore, dexamethasone alone is an appropriate alternative to VAD as a pretransplant induction therapy.

A recently completed Mayo Clinic study of 50 patients with previously untreated MM showed a response rate of 64% with the combination induction therapy of low-dose thalidomide (200 mg/d) and pulsed dexamethasone (40 mg on days 1–4, 9–12, 17–20 [odd cycles] and on days 1–4 [even cycles]) [52]. This regimen may be an alternative to VAD or dexamethasone alone as pretransplant induction therapy. An Eastern Cooperative Oncology Group randomized Phase III trial of thalidomide plus dexamethasone versus dexamethasone alone, as induction therapy for newly diagnosed MM, has just completed accrual in the US; results are expected in 2004.

Conditioning therapy and stem cell transplantation

The standard conditioning regimen for ASCT is melphalan at a dose of 200 mg/m^2. Total body irradiation has fallen out of favor following the results of a French randomized trial that showed an increase in toxicity with no significant survival benefit [53]. Similarly, stem cells are not purged of contaminating MM cells or enriched for CD34$^+$ cells, based on the results of a large randomized trial that showed no clinical benefit [54].

Single versus double transplantation

Barlogie et al. at the University of Arkansas in Little Rock, AR, USA, advocate the approach of tandem (double) ASCT to improve CR rates and survival time [55–58]. With tandem transplantation, patients receive a second planned transplant upon recovery from the first procedure. Using this approach, a study of 231 patients with newly diagnosed MM showed the median overall survival time to be greater than 5 years [59]. These results have prompted several studies of tandem ASCT in MM [60].

Preliminary data from four different randomized trials indicate a slight increase in response rates and possible improvement in event-free survival time with tandem transplantation [60]. To date, only one of the four trials (IFM 94) has shown significant improvement in overall survival [60,61]. In the IFM 94 trial the 7-year overall survival rate was 42% with a double transplant and 21% with a single transplant. Corresponding rates for event-free survival were 20% and 10%, respectively. The other trials have a shorter follow-up than IFM 94. The final results of these trials will hopefully determine whether tandem ASCT is superior to single ASCT. Whilst the role of tandem transplantation remains to be defined, it is reasonable to harvest enough stem cells for two transplants. At the Mayo Clinic, for example, a single transplant is carried out with half of the collected stem cells; the other half are cryopreserved for transplantation at relapse. A study by Sirohi et al. suggests that this strategy produces results equivalent to those reported with tandem transplantation [62].

Allogeneic transplantation (also see Chapter 5)

Allogeneic transplantation eliminates the problem of tumor cell contamination of the stem cells, which is inevitable with ASCT. Furthermore, there is evidence of a graft versus myeloma effect with allografting [63]. Allogeneic transplantation leads to prolonged disease-free survival in approximately 20% of patients [64,65]. The high treatment-related mortality rate (30%–50%) and significant toxicity from graft-versus-host disease (GvHD) have limited the role of this procedure in the treatment of MM [64,65]. As a result, conventional allogeneic stem cell transplantation is rarely recommended for the initial treatment of MM.

There is a growing interest in the study of non-myeloablative ("mini") allogeneic transplantation for selected patients with MM, either immediately following early ASCT [66] or at relapse.

Maloney et al. reported the results of 32 patients treated with ASCT followed by a non-myeloablative allogeneic transplantation [67]. Mycophenolate, cyclosporin, and total body irradiation (2 Gy) were used as conditioning agents for the non-myeloablative allogeneic transplantation. All allografts were from human leukocyte antigen-identical sibling donors. The response rate to therapy was 84%, with a relatively low day-100 treatment-related mortality rate of 6%. However, the high incidence of acute (45%) and chronic (55%) GvHD continues to limit enthusiasm for this approach. Until further refinements are made and additional confirmatory studies are completed, the role of non-myeloablative allogeneic stem cell transplantation in the treatment of MM must be considered investigational, and only conducted as part of clinical trials.

Maintenance therapy

The role of maintenance therapy following either conventional-dose melphalan–prednisone therapy or stem cell transplantation is investigational. Several studies have shown that IFN-α (usually 3 million units subcutaneously, three times a week) as maintenance therapy prolongs the plateau phase in MM [68–71]. Others have failed to show such an effect, and overall survival was not prolonged [72–74]. The Myeloma Trialists' Collaborative Group has completed a meta-analysis of maintenance therapy with IFN-α in MM [36]. The results demonstrated a slight increase in overall survival by about 4 months, but the benefit was restricted to the smaller trials. IFN-α therapy is also associated with adverse effects such as fever, muscle ache, flu-like illness, granulocytopenia, and fatigue. These effects, together with the cost and the minimal benefits of IFN-α, have impeded its routine use as a maintenance therapy.

Prednisone at low doses is more promising [75]. Presently, clinical trials are being designed to study the role of low-dose prednisone, thalidomide, dendritic cell vaccination, and other novel approaches in maintenance therapy following stem cell transplantation or conventional chemotherapy.

Treatment of relapsed or refractory myeloma

Approach to therapy

Current therapy for relapsed or refractory MM is inadequate because remissions with most regimens are short-lived. Typically, patients who relapse or are refractory to initial chemotherapy are treated with either second-line chemotherapy regimens (VAD, VBMCP), high-dose steroids (pulsed methylprednisolone or dexamethasone), bortezomib, or thalidomide. If the patient has had no significant exposure to alkylating agents (eg, no more than 6 months of melphalan treatment), or if cryopreserved stem cells are available, then ASCT must also be considered [76]. Another option is to enroll the patient in a clinical trial that is evaluating promising new agents.

The choice and sequence of therapy depends on several factors, including the nature of the relapse, response to initial therapy, number of prior treatment regimens, age, performance status, and patient preference.

In general, patients who relapse more than 6 months after alkylator-based therapy-induced remission should receive the same regimen. However, if the response duration following alkylator-based therapy is brief (<6 months) or the patient relapses shortly after stem cell transplantation, high-dose steroids may be a reasonable option. A second transplant is probably futile in patients who relapse early (<6 months) following the initial therapeutic procedure.

Patients with extensive prior therapy, advanced age, and poor performance status may not tolerate aggressive approaches such as ASCT or combination chemotherapy. In such patients, melphalan–prednisone, single-agent dexamethasone, or thalidomide are reasonable choices.

Newly diagnosed patients with good performance status who are refractory to VAD induction therapy or other induction regimens (eg, patients with primary refractory MM) do benefit from transplantation [48]. Depending on the clinical situation, these patients can either proceed directly to stem cell harvesting and transplantation without further therapy, or receive alternative induction regimens to try and achieve a response, thereby minimizing residual tumor volume at the time of harvesting and transplantation.

Therapeutic decisions are based on the risks and benefits of each option in conjunction with the patients' wishes. Patients refractory to one regimen may respond to another. Consideration must also be given to palliative and supportive care.

Thalidomide (also see Chapter 4)

The options available to patients with relapsed MM have increased with the renaissance of thalidomide – a drug with a notorious past due to its teratogenicity [77,78]. The activity of thalidomide in relapsed and refractory MM was first demonstrated by Singhal et al. at the University of Arkansas [79]. They observed a response rate of 32% in a group of heavily pre-treated patients, many of whom had failed two transplants. A study update confirmed these results and demonstrated 2-year overall and event-free survival rates of 48% and 20%, respectively [80]. Other groups have also confirmed the 25%–35% response rate seen with thalidomide in patients with relapsed and refractory MM. The median response duration is approximately 9–12 months [81–83].

The usual starting dose is 200 mg/d, increasing to 400 mg/d after 2 weeks. The majority of patients will respond to these dose levels, and further dose escalation is not usually needed. However, there may be occasional patients in whom a higher dose (up to 800 mg/d) is required to achieve or sustain a response.

Due to its severe teratogenicity, the use of thalidomide in pregnant women is absolutely contraindicated. In the US, all patients, physicians, and pharmacists must participate in the System for Thalidomide Education and Prescribing Safety (STEPS) program, which explains these risks and precautions, prior to

Common side effects	Less common side effects
Constipation	Bradycardia
Fatigue	Deep-vein thrombosis
Peripheral neuropathy	Edema
Sedation	Hyperglycemia
Skin rash	Hypoglycemia
	Hypothyroidism
	Impotence
	Increased liver enzyme levels
	Menstrual irregularities
	Neutropenia

Table 1. Side effects of thalidomide.

starting therapy [84]. The side effects of thalidomide are outlined in **Table 1**.

Since severe constipation is a common problem, laxatives are recommended prophylactically. If a skin rash occurs, the drug should be discontinued and restarted at a lower dose once the rash has cleared. Thalidomide can also cause peripheral neuropathy following chronic use over a period of several months.

Bortezomib (also see Chapter 3)

Bortezomib (formerly known as PS-341) is another active agent in refractory MM. Bortezomib is a selective inhibitor of the proteasome pathway, a critical pathway for the degradation of ubiquitinated proteins in the cell [85]. A recent multicenter trial of bortezomib in patients with refractory MM has shown a response rate of 32% [86]. The dose of bortezomib used in this trial was a 1.3 mg/m^2 intravenous push on days 1, 4, 8, and 11 of a 21-day cycle, for a total of 8 cycles. The main side effects were fatigue, cytopenia, neuropathy, and gastrointestinal symptoms. Based on the results of this trial, in May 2003 the US Food and Drug Administration gave accelerated approval for bortezomib in the treatment of refractory

MM in patients who have received at least two prior therapies and have demonstrated disease progression on the last therapy. A confirmatory Phase III trial comparing bortezomib with high-dose dexamethasone in the treatment of refractory MM has recently been completed.

Investigational therapy for relapsed/ refractory multiple myeloma

Given the activity of thalidomide in MM, investigations are in progress to identify a safer and more active analog. Immunomodulatory drugs (IMiDs) represent a class of thalidomide analogues that have shown promise in laboratory studies. Two Phase I trials with one of the IMiDs (CC-5013) have shown significant activity in heavily pretreated patients with refractory disease [87,88]. A recent Phase II confirmatory trial showed a preliminary response rate of 33% in the first 19 evaluable patients treated with CC-5013 [89]. Confirmatory Phase II and III trials with CC-5013 are ongoing.

Other active areas of investigation include dendritic cell vaccination, 2-methoxyestradiol, farnesyl transferase inhibitors, flavopiridol, and inhibitors of angiogenic cytokines.

Supportive care strategies

MM is characterized by lytic bony lesions, fractures, and osteoporosis, which all cause significant pain. Anemia, infections, hypercalcemia, and renal failure are other common complications. As a result, supportive care measures are important in management.

Prevention of bone disease (also see Chapter 6)

One of the goals of supportive care of MM patients is to reduce the incidence of lytic bone lesions and fractures. Recent studies have shown that the use of aminobisphosphonates (such as pamidronate or zoledronate) can delay or prevent lytic bone lesions, osteoporosis, and vertebral compression fractures [90]. Randomized trials show that intravenous pamidronate at a dose of

90 mg, administered over 4 hours every month, reduces skeletal complications and improves the quality of life of patients with MM [18,19]. Zoledronate is as effective as pamidronate, but has a much shorter infusion time of 15 minutes [20,21].

Based on these studies, it is now recommended that all patients with MM bone disease receive bisphosphonate therapy every month for an indefinite period of time. The role of bisphosphonates in patients who do not have any evidence of bone disease (eg, patients with SM) remains unclear and requires further study.

Treatment of anemia

Anemia is another major source of distress for patients with MM, resulting in fatigue and poor performance status. Reversible causes of anemia, such as iron, folate, or B_{12} deficiency, must be identified and treated. Anemia is often secondary to bone marrow involvement and renal dysfunction. Treatment of the underlying disease and improvement in renal function often leads to an increase in hemoglobin concentration. Erythropoietin therapy can improve the anemia associated with MM and is well tolerated [91,92]. It should be considered for MM patients with symptomatic anemia who are receiving myelosuppressive chemotherapy or who have significant renal dysfunction. Transfusions are indicated for patients with severe anemia who do not gain significant benefit from erythropoietin therapy.

Management of infections

Patients with MM are prone to infectious complications due to suppressed humoral and cell-mediated immunity, and the added effects of therapy. The following methods of management should be undertaken:

- Patients should be vaccinated against *Streptococcus pneumoniae* and *Hemophilus influenzae* – the principal organisms involved – though immune responses are attenuated in MM [93]. Administration of the annual influenza vaccine is also recommended.

- Patients with severe hypogammaglobulinemia and recurrent infections may benefit from monthly intravenous Ig infusions [94].
- Patients are prone to herpes zoster activation, so antiviral therapy is required to prevent dissemination.
- Patients receiving high-dose steroid regimens must be considered for prophylactic therapy against *Pneumocystis carinii* with trimethoprim-sulfamethoxazole [95].
- Patients receiving high-dose steroid therapy can also incur fungal infections, but serious infections are rare and there are no data on the role of antifungal prophylaxis.

A large randomized trial by the Eastern Cooperative Oncology Group is currently in progress to determine the role of prophylactic antibiotics in the treatment of MM patients who are undergoing chemotherapy.

Management of renal failure

Patients with MM are prone to renal failure from a variety of causes and should, therefore, avoid exposure to nephrotoxic drugs. In addition, exposure to radiographic contrast media should be limited, though the risk of renal toxicity is small provided that patients are adequately hydrated. Prompt treatment of MM with chemotherapy is critical for the control of renal failure [96].

Hypercalcemia

The most common reversible causes of renal failure in MM are hypercalcemia and dehydration. Hypercalcemia is a consequence of increased bone resorption mediated by cytokines. The current treatment of hypercalcemia in MM is aggressive hydration and corticosteroid therapy. Bisphosphonates should be given if there is no response to therapy or if the hypercalcemia is severe. A single intravenous dose of pamidronate (60–90 mg over 2–4 hours) will normalize the calcium levels within 24–72 hours in most patients [97]. Zoledronate (4 mg intravenously over 15 minutes) may be more potent than pamidronate in the treatment of hypercalcemia, and is a good alternative [98]. With the advent of bisphosphonates, true refractory hypercalcemia is rare. If a rapid reduction in serum calcium is needed, salmon calcitonin (4 units/kg every 12 hours) is occasionally used. However, a skin test (0.1 mL of a 10 units/mL dilution intracutaneously) is performed prior to administering salmon calcitonin to rule out hypersensitivity. Agents such as mithramycin and gallium nitrate are no longer used routinely for the management of hypercalcemia.

Dehydration

Dehydration in MM is usually seen in the setting of hypercalcemia, but is an important contributor to renal failure. Adequate hydration along with treatment of hypercalcemia and prompt initiation of specific antimyeloma therapy can help reverse renal failure.

Light-chain cast nephropathy

Light-chain cast nephropathy (myeloma kidney) is an important cause of renal failure, and requires treatment with hydration and institution of chemotherapy to control the light-chain production. Alkaline diuresis can be helpful by limiting the precipitation of casts. Selected patients with excess light-chain excretion in the urine and evolving acute renal failure due to cast nephropathy may benefit from plasmapheresis. Data from a small randomized trial demonstrated that plasmapheresis can lead to recovery of renal function [99].

Pain control measures

Most patients experience an improvement in symptoms with the initiation of specific chemotherapy. However, appropriate pain-control measures are often required until the disease is controlled. Some patients need hospitalization for pain control. Bone pain caused by lytic lesions or fractures may be relieved by narcotic analgesics. Alternatively, splinting or other orthopedic interventions such as vertebroplasty can reduce pain. Physical therapy and activity should be encouraged: in the first 6 months following MM diagnosis there is a high risk of deep-vein thrombosis, which is a likely result of immobilization.

Reducing mild pain

Mild degrees of pain can be controlled with acetaminophen-codeine, acetaminophen-oxycodone, or similar analgesic preparations. However, dose escalation for controlling more severe pain is prevented by the amount of acetaminophen in these preparations, which confers the risk of acetaminophen hepatotoxicity. Nonsteroidal anti-inflammatory agents, which can also be used to reduce mild pain, can precipitate renal failure or exaggerate steroid-induced gastritis in MM and should generally be avoided [100,101].

Reducing severe pain

For severe pain, oral morphine sulfate is effective. It is administered as a sustained-release preparation, with an immediate-release form available for breakthrough pain. Alternatives to morphine include hydromorphone or transdermal fentanyl. Radiation therapy to limited areas involved by myeloma is indicated to control pain that is refractory to narcotics. It may also be used to prevent or treat spinal cord compression. Orthopedic interventions and/or radiation may be needed to prevent or treat pathologic fracture in susceptible long bones with large lytic lesions. In general, it is wise to limit the amount of radiation that is administered, since radiation to large areas of bone can subsequently limit the amount of systemic chemotherapy that can be administered. The dose of radiation used needs to be individualized; some patients may require doses of less than the traditional 30 Gy administered in 10 fractions [102].

Future directions

Several novel agents and strategies have emerged for the treatment of MM. Furthermore, non-myeloablative allogeneic transplantation appears promising. Based on these strategies, the approach to management of MM and supportive care will continue to evolve. One goal will be to incorporate novel agents into initial therapy in a way that limits or prevents the need for transplantation. Another goal will be to develop effective maintenance therapy that will delay relapse. The eventual goal is a cure.

Acknowledgements

Supported in part by Grants CA 100080, CA 93842, CA85818, and CA62242 from the National Cancer Institute, MD, USA. Dr Rajkumar is a Leukemia and Lymphoma Society of America Translational Research Awardee and is also supported by the Goldman Philanthropic Partnerships, IL, USA, and the Multiple Myeloma Research Foundation, CT, USA.

References

1. Rajkumar SV, Kyle RA. *Management of Patients With Asymptomatic or Newly Diagnosed Myeloma: Understanding the Disease and Update on Novel Treatment Approaches*. Philadelphia, PA: Seton Hall University School of Graduate Medical Education, American Academy of CME, and Omegamed, Inc., 2002.
2. Rajkumar SV, Dispenzieri A, Fonseca R et al. Thalidomide for previously untreated indolent or smoldering multiple myeloma. *Leukemia* 2001;15:1274–6.
3. Kyle RA. "Benign" monoclonal gammopathy – after 20 to 35 years of follow-up. *Mayo Clin Proc* 1993;68:26–36.
4. Kyle RA, Therneau TM, Rajkumar SV et al. A long-term study of prognosis in monoclonal gammopathy of undetermined significance. *N Engl J Med* 2002;346:564–9.
5. Cesana C, Klersy C, Barbarano L et al. Prognostic factors for malignant transformation in monoclonal gammopathy of undetermined significance and smoldering multiple myeloma. *J Clin Oncol* 2002;20:1625–34.
6. Greipp PR, Kyle RA. Staging, kinetics, and prognosis of multiple myeloma. In: Wiernik PH, Canellos GP, Dutcher JP et al., editors. *Neoplastic Diseases of the Blood*. New York, NY: Churchill Livingstone, 1996:537–59.
7. Kyle RA, Greipp PR. Smoldering multiple myeloma. *N Engl J Med* 1980;302:1347–9.
8. Witzig TE, Kyle RA, O'Fallon WM et al. Detection of peripheral blood plasma cells as a predictor of disease course in patients with smouldering multiple myeloma. *Br J Haematol* 1994;87:266–72.
9. Weber DM, Dimopoulos MA, Moulopoulos LA et al. Prognostic features of asymptomatic multiple myeloma. *Br J Haematol* 1997;97:810–4.
10. Dimopoulos MA, Moulopoulos LA, Maniatis A et al. Solitary plasmacytoma of bone and asymptomatic multiple myeloma. *Blood* 2000;96:2037–44.
11. Dimopoulos MA, Moulopoulos A, Smith T et al. Risk of disease progression in asymptomatic multiple myeloma. *Am J Med* 1993;94:57–61.

12. Greipp PR, Kyle RA. Clinical, morphological, and cell kinetic differences among multiple myeloma, monoclonal gammopathy of undetermined significance, and smoldering multiple myeloma. *Blood* 1983;62:166–71.
13. Hjorth M, Hellquist L, Holmberg E et al. Initial versus deferred melphalan-prednisone therapy for asymptomatic multiple myeloma stage I – a randomized study. Myeloma Group of Western Sweden. *Eur J Haematol* 1993;50:95–102.
14. Rajkumar SV, Hayman S, Fonseca R et al. Thalidomide plus dexamethasone (thal/dex) and thalidomide alone (Thal) as first line therapy for newly diagnosed myeloma (MM). *Blood* 2000;96:168A (Abstr.).
15. Weber DM, Rankin K, Gavino M et al. Angiogenesis factors and sensitivity to thalidomide in previously untreated multiple myeloma (MM). *Blood* 2000;96:168A (Abstr.).
16. Rajkumar SV, Dispenzieri A, Fonseca R et al. Thalidomide for previously untreated indolent or smoldering multiple myeloma. *Leukemia* 2001;15:1274–76.
17. Rajkumar SV, Gertz MA, Lacy MQ et al. Thalidomide as initial therapy for early-stage myeloma. *Leukemia* 2003;17:775–9.
18. Berenson JR, Lichtenstein A, Porter L et al. Efficacy of pamidronate in reducing skeletal events in patients with advanced multiple myeloma. Myeloma Aredia Study Group. *N Engl J Med* 1996;334:488–93.
19. Berenson JR, Lichtenstein A, Porter L et al. Long-term pamidronate treatment of advanced multiple myeloma patients reduces skeletal events. Myeloma Aredia Study Group. *J Clin Oncol* 1998;16:593–602.
20. Rosen LS, Gordon D, Antonio BS et al. Zoledronic acid versus pamidronate in the treatment of skeletal metastases in patients with breast cancer or osteolytic lesions of multiple myeloma: a phase III, double blind, comparative trial. *Cancer J* 2001;7:377–87.
21. Berenson JR, Rosen LS, Howell A et al. Zoledronic acid reduces skeletal-related events in patients with osteolytic metastases. [Published erratum appears in *Cancer* 2001;91:1956]. *Cancer* 2001;91:1191–200.
22. Dimopoulos MA, Moulopoulos LA, Maniatis A et al. Solitary plasmacytoma of bone and asymptomatic multiple myeloma. *Blood* 2000;96:2037–44.
23. Dimopoulos MA, Kiamouris C, Moulopoulos LA. Solitary plasmacytoma of bone and extramedullary plasmacytoma. *Hematol Oncol Clin North Am* 1999;13:1249–57.
24. Wilder RB, Ha CH, Cox JD et al. Persistence of myeloma protein for more than 1 year after radiotherapy is an adverse prognostic factor in solitary plasmacytoma of bone. *Cancer* 2002;94:1532–7.
25. Kumar S, Fonseca R, Dispenzieri A et al. Prognostic value of angiogenesis in solitary bone plasmacytoma. *Blood* 2003;101:1715–7.
26. Gertz MA, Rajkumar SV. Primary systemic amyloidosis. *Curr Treat Options Oncol* 2002;3:261–71.
27. Falk RH, Comenzo RL, Skinner M. The systemic amyloidoses [see comments]. *N Engl J Med* 1997;337:898–909. Comment in: *N Engl J Med* 1998;338:264–5.
28. Kyle RA, Gertz MA, Greipp PR et al. A trial of three regimens for primary amyloidosis: colchicine alone, melphalan and prednisone, and melphalan, prednisone, and colchicine [see comment]. *N Engl J Med* 1997;336:1202–7. Comment in: *ACP J Club* 1997;127(3):71.
29. Comenzo RL, Gertz MA. Autologous stem cell transplantation for primary systemic amyloidosis. *Blood* 2002;99:4276–82.
30. Attal M, Harousseau JL, Stoppa AM et al. A prospective, randomized trial of autologous bone marrow transplantation and chemotherapy in multiple myeloma. Intergroupe Francais du Myelome. *N Engl J Med* 1996;335:91–7.

31. Child JA, Morgan GJ, Davies FE et al. High-dose chemotherapy with hematopoietic stem-cell rescue for multiple myeloma. *N Engl J Med* 2003;348:1875–83.
32. Myeloma Trialists' Collaborative Group. Combination chemotherapy versus melphalan plus prednisone as treatment for multiple myeloma: an overview of 6,633 patients from 27 randomized trials. *J Clin Oncol* 1998;16:3832–42.
33. Kovacsovics TJ, Delaly A. Intensive treatment strategies in multiple myeloma. *Semin Hematol* 1997;34(1 Suppl. 1):49–60.
34. Alexanian R, Dimopoulos M. The treatment of multiple myeloma. *New Engl J Med* 1994;330:484–9.
35. Oken MM, Harrington DP, Abramson N et al. Comparison of melphalan and prednisone with vincristine, carmustine, melphalan, cyclophosphamide, and prednisone in the treatment of multiple myeloma: results of Eastern Cooperative Oncology Group Study E2479. *Cancer* 1997;79:1561–7.
36. The Myeloma Trialists' Collaborative Group. Interferon as therapy for multiple myeloma: an individual patient data overview of 24 randomized trials and 4012 patients. *Br J Haematol* 2001;113:1020–34.
37. Harousseau JL, Attal M. The role of autologous hematopoietic stem cell transplantation in multiple myeloma. *Semin Hematol* 1997;34(1 Suppl. 1):61–6.
38. Barlogie B, Jagannath S, Epstein J et al. Biology and therapy of multiple myeloma in 1996. *Semin Hematol* 1997;34(1 Suppl. 1):67–72.
39. Gertz MA, Pineda AA, Chen MG et al. Refractory and relapsing multiple myeloma treated by blood stem cell transplantation. *Am J Med Sci* 1995;309:152–61.
40. Child JA, Morgan GJ, Davies FE et al. High-dose chemotherapy with hematopoietic stem-cell rescue for multiple myeloma. *N Engl J Med* 2003;348:1875–83.
41. Bladé J, Sureda A, Ribera JM et al. High-dose therapy autotransplantation/intensification vs continued conventional chemotherapy in multiple myeloma patients responding to initial treatment chemotherapy. Results of a Prospective Randomized Trial from the Spanish Cooperative Group PETHEMA. *Blood* 2001;98:815A (Abstr.).
42. Siegel DS, Desikan KR, Mehta J et al. Age is not a prognostic variable with autotransplants for multiple myeloma. *Blood* 1999;93:51–4.
43. Fermand JP, Ravaud P, Chevret S et al. High-dose therapy and autologous peripheral blood stem cell transplantation in multiple myeloma: up-front or rescue treatment? Results of a multicenter sequential randomized clinical trial. *Blood* 1998;92:3131–6.
44. Fermand JP, Ravaud P, Chevret S et al. Early versus late high dose therapy (HDT) and autologous peripheral blood stem cell (PBSC) transplantation in multiple myeloma (MM): results of a prospective randomized trial. *Blood* 1996;88(Suppl. 1):685A (Abstr.).
45. Facon T, Mary JY, Harousseau JL et al. Front-line or rescue autologous bone marrow transplantation (ABMT) following a first course of high dose melphalan (HDM) in multiple myeloma (MM). Preliminary results of a prospective randomized trial (CIAM protocol). *Blood* 1996;88(Suppl. 1):685A (Abstr.).
46. Alexanian R, Barlogie B, Tucker S. VAD-based regimens as primary treatment for multiple myeloma. *Am J Hematol* 1990;33:86–9.
47. Anderson H, Scarffe JH, Ranson M et al. VAD chemotherapy as remission induction for multiple myeloma. *Br J Cancer* 1995;71:326–30.
48. Rajkumar SV, Fonseca R, Lacy MQ et al. Autologous stem cell transplantation for relapsed and primary refractory myeloma. *Bone Marrow Transplant* 1999;23:1267–72.
49. Singhal S, Powles R, Sirohi B et al. Response to induction chemotherapy is not essential to obtain survival benefit from high-dose melphalan and autotransplantation in myeloma. *Blood* 2001;98:816A (Abstr.).

50. Alexanian R, Dimopoulos MA, Delasalle K et al. Primary dexamethasone treatment of multiple myeloma. *Blood* 1992;80:887–90.
51. Anagnostopoulos A, Aleman A, Williams P et al. Autologous stem cell transplantation (ASCT) after nonmyelosuppressive induction therapy with dexamethasone alone is safe and effective for newly diagnosed multiple myeloma (MM) pts who receive high-dose chemotherapy (HDC). *Blood* 2001;98:683A (Abstr.).
52. Rajkumar SV, Hayman S, Gertz MA et al. Combination therapy with thalidomide plus dexamethasone for newly diagnosed myeloma. *J Clin Oncol* 2002;20:4319–23.
53. Moreau P, Facon T, Attal M et al. Comparison of 200 mg/m^2 melphalan and 8 Gy total body irradiation plus 140 mg/m^2 melphalan as conditioning regimens for peripheral blood stem cell transplantation in patients with newly diagnosed multiple myeloma: final analysis of the Intergroupe Francophone du Myélome 9502 randomized trial. *Blood* 2002;99:731–5.
54. Stewart AK, Vescio R, Schiller G et al. Purging of autologous peripheral-blood stem cells using CD34 selection does not improve overall or progression-free survival after high-dose chemotherapy for multiple myeloma: results of a multicenter randomized controlled trial. *J Clin Oncol* 2001;19:3771–9.
55. Barlogie B, Jagannath S, Vesole DH et al. Superiority of tandem autologous transplantation over standard therapy for previously untreated multiple myeloma. *Blood* 1997;89:789–93.
56. Vesole DH, Barlogie B, Jagannath S et al. High-dose therapy for refractory multiple myeloma: improved prognosis with better supportive care and double transplants. *Blood* 1994;84:950–6.
57. Tricot G, Jagannath S, Vesole DH et al. Hematopoietic stem cell transplants for multiple myeloma. *Leuk Lymphoma* 1996;22:25–36.
58. Desikan R, Barlogie B, Sawyer J et al. Results of high-dose therapy for 1000 patients with multiple myeloma: durable complete remissions and superior survival in the absence of chromosome 13 abnormalities. *Blood* 2000;95:4008–10.
59. Barlogie B, Jagannath S, Desikan KR et al. Total therapy with tandem transplants for newly diagnosed multiple myeloma. *Blood* 1999;93:55–65.
60. Dalton WS, Bergsagel PL, Kuehl WM et al. Multiple myeloma. In: Schechter GP, Broudy VB, Williams ME, editors. *Hematology 2001*. Washington, DC: American Society of Hematology, 2001:157–77.
61. Attal M, Harousseau JL, Facon T et al. Double autologous transplantation improves survival of multiple myeloma patients: final analysis of a prospective randomized study of the "Intergroupe Francophone du Myelome" (IFM 94). *Blood* 2002;100:5A (Abstr.).
62. Sirohi B, Powles R, Singhal S et al. High-dose melphalan and second autografts for myeloma relapsing after one autograft: results equivalent to tandem autotransplantation. *Blood* 2001;98:402A (Abstr.).
63. Tricot G, Vesole DH, Jagannath S et al. Graft-versus-myeloma effect: proof of principle. *Blood* 1996;87:1196–8.
64. Bensinger WI, Buckner CD, Anasetti C et al. Allogeneic marrow transplantation for multiple myeloma: an analysis of risk factors on outcome. *Blood* 1996;88:2787–93.
65. Cavo M, Bandini G, Benni M et al. High-dose busulfan and cyclophosphamide are an effective conditioning regimen for allogeneic bone marrow transplantation in chemosensitive multiple myeloma. *Bone Marrow Transplant* 1998;22:27–32.
66. Molina A, Sahebi F, Maloney DG et al. Non-myeloablative peripheral blood stem cell (PBSC) allografts following cytoreductive autotransplants for treatment of multiple myeloma (MM). *Blood* 2000;96:480A (Abstr.).
67. Maloney DG, Sahebi F, Stockerl-Goldstein KE et al. Combining an allogeneic graft-vs-myeloma effect with high-dose autologous stem cell rescue in the treatment of multiple myeloma. *Blood* 2001;98:434A (Abstr.).

68. Shustik C. Interferon in the treatment of multiple myeloma. *Cancer Control* 1998;5:226–34.
69. Mandelli F, Avvisati G, Amadori S et al. Maintenance treatment with recombinant interferon alfa-2b in patients with multiple myeloma responding to conventional induction chemotherapy. *N Engl J Med* 1990;322:1430–4.
70. Browman GP, Bergsagel D, Sicheri D et al. Randomized trial of interferon maintenance in multiple myeloma: a study of the National Cancer Institute of Canada Clinical Trials Group. *J Clin Oncol* 1995;13:2354–60.
71. Westin J, Rodjer S, Turesson I et al. Interferon alfa-2b versus no maintenance therapy during the plateau phase in multiple myeloma: a randomized study. Cooperative Study Group. *Br J Haematol* 1995;89:561–8.
72. Salmon SE, Crowley JJ, Grogan TM et al. Combination chemotherapy, glucocorticoids, and interferon alfa in the treatment of multiple myeloma: a Southwest Oncology Group study. *J Clin Oncol* 1994;12:2405–14.
73. Peest D, Deicher H, Coldewey R et al. A comparison of polychemotherapy and melphalan/prednisone for primary remission induction, and interferon-alpha for maintenance treatment, in multiple myeloma. A prospective trial of the German Myeloma Treatment Group. *Eur J Cancer* 1995;31A:146–51.
74. Ludwig H, Cohen AM, Polliack A et al. Interferon-alpha for induction and maintenance in multiple myeloma: results of two multicenter randomized trials and summary of other studies. *Ann Oncol* 1995;6:467–76.
75. Salmon SE, Crowley JJ, Balcerzak SP et al. Interferon versus interferon plus prednisone remission maintenance therapy for multiple myeloma: a Southwest Oncology Group Study. *J Clin Oncol* 1998;16:890–6.
76. Vesole DH, Crowley JJ, Catchatourian R et al. High-dose melphalan with autotransplantation for refractory multiple myeloma: results of a Southwest Oncology Group phase II trial. *J Clin Oncol* 1999;17:2173–9.
77. Rajkumar SV, Witzig TE. A review of angiogenesis and antiangiogenic therapy with thalidomide in multiple myeloma. *Cancer Treat Rev* 2000;26:351–62.
78. Rajkumar SV, Kyle RA. Thalidomide in the treatment of plasma cell malignancies. *J Clin Oncol* 2001;19:3593–5.
79. Singhal S, Mehta J, Desikan R et al. Antitumor activity of thalidomide in refractory multiple myeloma. *New Engl J Med* 1999;341:1565–71.
80. Barlogie B, Spencer T, Tricot G et al. Long term follow up of 169 patients receiving a phase II trial of single agent thalidomide for advanced and refractory multiple myeloma (MM). *Blood* 2000;96:514A (Abstr.).
81. Rajkumar SV, Fonseca R, Dispenzieri A et al. Thalidomide in the treatment of relapsed multiple myeloma. *Mayo Clin Proc* 2000;75:897–901.
82. Rajkumar SV. Current status of thalidomide in the treatment of cancer. *Oncology (Huntingt)* 2001;15:867–74; discussion 877–9.
83. Kumar S, Gertz MA, Dispenzieri A et al. Response rate, durability of response, and survival after thalidomide therapy for relapsed multiple myeloma [see comment]. *Mayo Clin Proc* 2003;78:34–9. Comment in: *Mayo Clin Proc* 2003;78:15–7.
84. Hideshima T, Richardson P, Chauhan D et al. The proteasome inhibitor PS-341 inhibits growth, induces apoptosis, and overcomes drug resistance in human multiple myeloma cells. *Cancer Res* 2001;61:3071–6.
85. Zeldis JB, Williams BA, Thomas SD et al. S.T.E.P.S.: a comprehensive program for controlling and monitoring access to thalidomide. *Clin Ther* 1999;21:319–30.
86. Richardson PG, Barlogie B, Berenson J et al. A phase 2 study of bortezomib in relapsed refractory myeloma. *N Engl J Med* 2003;348:2609–17.

87. Richardson PG, Schlossman RL, Weller E et al. Immunomodulatory drug CC-5013 overcomes drug resistance and is well tolerated in patients with relapsed multiple myeloma. *Blood* 2002;100:3063–7.
88. Zangari M, Tricot G, Zeldis J et al. Results of phase I study of CC-5013 for the treatment of multiple myeloma (MM) patients who relapse after high dose chemotherapy (HDCT). *Blood* 2001;98:775A (Abstr.).
89. Richardson PG, Jagannath S, Schlossman RL et al. A multi-center, randomized, phase II study to evaluate the efficacy and safety of two CDC-5013 dose regimens when used alone or in combination with dexamethasone for the treatment of relapsed or refractory multiple myeloma. *Blood* 2002;100:104A (Abstr. 386).
90. Kyle RA. The role of bisphosphonates in multiple myeloma. *Ann Intern Med* 2000;132:734–6.
91. Mittelman M, Zeidman A, Fradin Z et al. Recombinant human erythropoietin in the treatment of multiple myeloma-associated anemia. *Acta Haematol* 1997;98:204–10.
92. Musto P, Falcone A, D'Arena G et al. Clinical results of recombinant erythropoietin in transfusion-dependent patients with refractory multiple myeloma: role of cytokines and monitoring of erythropoiesis. *Eur J Haematol* 1997;58:314–9.
93. Kelleher P, Chapel H. Infections: Principles of prevention and therapy. In: Mehta J, Singhal S, editors. *Myeloma*. London: Martin Dunitz Publishers, 2002:223–39.
94. Chapel HM, Lee M, Hargreaves R et al. Randomised trial of intravenous immunoglobulin as prophylaxis against infection in plateau-phase multiple myeloma. The UK Group for Immunoglobulin Replacement Therapy in Multiple Myeloma. *Lancet* 1994;343:1059–63.
95. van der Lelie J, Venema D, Kuijper EJ et al. *Pneumocystis carinii* pneumonia in HIV-negative patients with haematologic disease. *Infection* 1997;25:78–81.
96. Alexanian R, Barlogie B, Dixon D. Renal failure in multiple myeloma. Pathogenesis and prognostic implications. *Arch Intern Med* 1990;150:1693–5.
97. Gucalp R, Theriault R, Gill I et al. Treatment of cancer-associated hypercalcemia. Double-blind comparison of rapid and slow intravenous infusion regimens of pamidronate disodium and saline alone. *Arch Intern Med* 1994;154:1935–44.
98. Major P, Lortholary A, Hon J et al. Zoledronic acid is superior to pamidronate in the treatment of hypercalcemia of malignancy: a pooled analysis of two randomized, controlled clinical trials. *J Clin Oncol* 2001;19:558–67.
99. Johnson WJ, Kyle RA, Pineda AA et al. Treatment of renal failure associated with multiple myeloma. Plasmapheresis, hemodialysis, and chemotherapy. *Arch Intern Med* 1990;150:863–9.
100. Yussim E, Schwartz E, Sidi Y et al. Acute renal failure precipitated by non-steroidal anti-inflammatory drugs (NSAIDs) in multiple myeloma. *Am J Hematol* 1998;58:142–4.
101. Wu MJ, Kumar KS, Kulkarni G et al. Multiple myeloma in naproxen-induced acute renal failure. *N Engl J Med* 1987;317:170–1.
102. Shrieve DC. The role of radiotherapy. In: Mehta J, Singhal S, editors. *Myeloma*. London: Martin Dunitz Publishers, 2002:367–83.

Abbreviations

2ME2	2-methoxyestradiol
ABMT	autologous bone marrow transplantation
AL	amyloidosis
APL	acute promyelocytic leukemia
Apo2L	Apo2 ligand
ASCO	American Society of Clinical Oncology
ASCT	autologous stem cell transplantation
As_2O_3	arsenic trioxide
ATRA	all-*trans*-retinoic acid
BCRP	breast cancer resistance protein
BEAM	carmustine, etoposide, cytarabine, and melphalan
bFGF	basic fibroblast growth factor
BM	bone marrow
BMSC	bone marrow stromal cell
BP	non-nitrogen-containing bisphosphonate
BVAP	carmustine, vincristine, doxorubicin, and prednisone
CAMs	cell adhesion molecules
CAM-DR	cell adhesion-mediated drug resistance
CBV	cyclophosphamide, carmustine, and etoposide
CC	conventional chemotherapy
$cFLIP_L$	cellular FLICE-like inhibitory protein-long
CHOP	cyclophosphamide, hydroxydaunomycin, vincristine, and prednisone
CR	complete response/remission
DCEP	dexamethasone, cyclophosphamide, etoposide, and cisplatin
DLI	donor lymphocyte infusion

dPyr	deoxypyridinoline
DT-PACE	dexamethasone, thalidomide, cisplatin, doxorubicin, cyclophosphamide, and etoposide
EBMT	European Group for Blood and Marrow Transplantation
ECM	extracellular matrix
EFS	event-free survival
ERK	extracellular signal-regulated kinase
FasL	Fas ligand
FDA	US Food and Drug Administration
FGFR3	fibroblast growth factor receptor 3
FISH	fluorescence *in situ* hybridization
FLICE	Fas-associated death domain-like interleukin-1β-converting enzyme
FLIP	FLICE inhibitor protein
FN	fibronectin
FPP	farnesyl diphosphate
FTI	farnesyl transferase inhibitor
GA	geldanamycin
GC	glucocorticoid
γ-GCS	γ-glutamylcysteine synthase
GGTI	geranylgeranyl transferase inhibitor
GI	gastrointestinal
GR	glucocorticoid receptor
GSH	glutathione
GST	glutathione S-transferase
GvHD	graft versus host disease
GVM	graft versus myeloma
HBD	hormone-binding domain
HCV	hepatitis C virus
HDT	high-dose chemotherapy
HMCL	human myeloma cell lines
Hsp	heat shock protein
IAP	inhibitor of apoptosis
ICTP	carboxy-terminal telopeptide of type I collagen
IFM	Intergroupe Francophone du Myelome
IFN-α	interferon-α

Ig	immunoglobulin
IgAγ	immunoglobulin A gamma
IGF	insulin-like growth factor
IL	interleukin
IMiDs	immunomodulatory drugs
IR	ionizing radiation
JAK	Janus kinase
JNK	c-Jun N-terminal kinase
LAK	lymphokine-activated killer
L-PAM	L-phenylalanine mustard (melphalan)
LRP	lung resistance protein
LT	lymphotoxin
M	monoclonal
MAPK	mitogen-activated protein kinase
MAPKK	mitogen-activated protein kinase kinase (MEK)
MDR	multidrug resistance
MEK	mitogen-activated protein kinase kinase (MAPKK)
MGUS	monoclonal gammopathy of undetermined significance
MIP-1α	macrophage inflammatory protein-1α
MM	multiple myeloma
MRC	Medical Research Council
MRI	magnetic resonance imaging
MRP	multidrug resistance protein
N-BP	nitrogen-containing bisphosphonate
NF-κB	nuclear factor-κB
NK	natural killer
OPG	osteoprotegerin
OS	overall survival
PARP	poly(ADP-ribose) polymerase
PBSC	peripheral blood stem cell
PCD	programmed cell death
P-gp	P-glycoprotein
PI	phosphatidylinositol
PKC	protein kinase C
PML	promyelocytic leukemia
PR	partial response/remission

Pyr	pyridinoline
RAFTK	related focal adhesion tyrosine kinase
RANK	receptor activator of nuclear factor-κB
RANKL	RANK ligand
RB	retinoblastoma
SAHA	suberoylanilide hydroxamic acid
SCID	severe combined immunodeficiency
SCT	stem cell transplantation
SDF-1α	stromal-cell-derived factor-1α
SEER	Surveillance, Epidemiology, and End Results
SHP-2	SH2-containing protein tyrosine phosphatase
Smac	second mitochondria-derived activator of caspase
SM	smoldering myeloma
STAT	signal transducer and activator of transcription
STEPS	System for Thalidomide Education and Prescribing Safety
TBI	total body irradiation
TGF-β	tumor growth factor-β
Thal	thalidomide
TNF-α	tumor necrosis factor-α
topo	topoisomerase
TRAIL	tumor necrosis factor-related apoptosis-inducing ligand
VAD	vincristine, doxorubicin, and pulsed dexamethasone
VAMP	vinblastine, doxorubicin, methotrexate, and prednisone
VBMCP	vincristine, carmustine (BCNU), melphalan, cyclophosphamide, and prednisone
VEGF	vascular endothelial growth factor
VMCP	vincristine, melphalan, cyclophosphamide, and prednisone
XIAP	X-linked inhibitor of apoptosis protein

Index

References to figures are in **bold**
References to tables are in *italics*

B

D

H

J

K

L

M

Q

R

S